Praise for
Unprocessed Living

Hear from my clients and friends who have removed processed foods from their diet:

"I removed a large amount of processed food from my diet, and as a result, I feel healthier and better about what I'm putting in my body. By using the principles in this book, I stopped eating foods with ingredients I couldn't pronounce or were horrible for me. I know I'm creating a healthier future for my family. I used to have headaches and after I removed diet sodas, I rarely get them anymore."

—Becca R., Lexington, KY

"I removed white flour and sugar from my diet, and as a result, I lost 12 pounds and feel like I did 20 years ago. I have so much more energy, it's really unbelievable. I also added 64 ounces of water and/ or plain tea daily and my sugar cravings and appetite has decreased. I noticed my skin, hair and nails are healthier than before as well."

—Karen B., Northern VA

"Being tired, overweight, sore and in pain wa _____ Finally, I'd had enough and made the commitment to take processed foods out of my diet. At first it was very hard—almost everything in our family's diet consisted of processed foods. Slowly we eliminated more and more processed foods, but after educating ourselves on what a healthy lifestyle looks like, now even my kids read labels at the store. It's been 14 months and I'm proud to say we've cut out an impressive amount of packaged and processed foods. Cooking at home isn't hard since we've gotten used to pre-planning our meals.

"One great example that even the kids were shocked about were the ingredients on the birthday cakes you buy at the grocery store— we couldn't even pronounce almost every ingredient. Making meals and even treats at home (cakes, ice cream, donuts) and regular foods without cans or boxes is cheaper and tastes just as delicious.

"While we'd love to shop at farmer's markets or specialty stores—being a busy family it's a little tough—we've gotten great at shopping at all the regular grocery stores to get what's healthy. Some days it's hard and we're not perfect—but trying is the most important.

"Now 14 months later, in addition to my 75-pound weight loss and my family feeling healthier and happier, my hair doesn't fall out every time I brush it, my adult acne is gone, daily joint and back pain is non-existent and sleeping is even better. My kids' attitudes, sleep and school work has all also improved. I can't imagine going back to the way we used to eat."

—Jennifer B., Northern VA

"I removed all processed foods, sugar and dairy from my diet for one month, and as a result, I lost 10 pounds in that month and feel more energized, positive and focused. Needless to say, it's a no-brainer that I will continue eating this way!"

—Robin K., Worchester, MA

"I have lost over 20 pounds and several inches since I started coming to Cindy's classes. I certainly feel healthy and more energetic when I keep processed foods out of my diet. Cindy has provided me with such a comprehensive and extensive body of knowledge."

—Pat L, Northern VA

"By using the swap lists in this book, I stopped eating white flours, sugars and other processed foods and I don't have arthritis pain in my joints anymore."

—Beth T., Northern VA

"I was fortunate enough to attend several of Cindy's clean eating workshops at my Over 55 Community. As a result of gradually including recommendations related to cooking oils and unprocessed foods to exclude from my diet, this Senior Citizen has lost 25 pounds and decreased my Type 2 Diabetes medications from 5 to 2 prescriptions!"

—Chris P., Northern VA

"By using the steps in this book, I have become a more conscientious cook and consumer, ever mindful to choose healthier foods and products."

—Diane A., Northern VA

"Cindy's book is simple and easy to follow. She shows you how to transition your family away from processed foods to begin the journey back toward better health and vitality."

—Terry Wahls M.D., author of the bestseller *The Wahls Protocol: A Radical New Way to Treat All Chronic Autoimmune Conditions Using Paleo Principles*

"With Unprocessed Living, you'll learn how to critically read food labels, substitute processed ingredients for healthier alternatives, create shopping lists and meal plans, stock your pantry and fridge, save time and money in the kitchen, eat out, navigate picky kids, find alternatives for school, sports, holidays, and household items like laundry soap, as well as tons of recipes to get you started.... In other words, it's all here! Cindy has all the bases covered to get you and your family on the track to real food and better health!"

—Sarah Ballantyne, PhD, New York Times bestselling author of *The Paleo Approach* and *The Paleo Approach Cookbook*

Unprocessed Living

3 Easy Steps to Transition into Healthy Eating

By Cindy Santa Ana, CHC

To contact the author, visit www.UnlockBetterHealth.com

ISBN: 978–0-692–39514–1

Printed in the United States of America

Cover photo by Roosh Benham, Roosh Photography.
Back cover photo by Olivia Pisaretz Photography.

Dedication:

To every woman looking to create a healthy, happy home life for her family.

Contents

Foreword by Dr. Josh Axe

As an advocate for holistic, natural medicine, I see food as a healing mechanism. Science today has discovered that the food we eat can hurt or heal us and the quality of our food counts. But knowing how to source, prepare and serve healthy food to our families can be a challenge. Cindy has given us the tools to achieve this in her new book, *Unprocessed Living*.

Cindy provides detailed information on deciphering confusing food labels and provides healthier alternatives to the processed foods we've grown accustomed to eating. She teaches you how to stock your pantry and fridge with healthy foods that will nurture your body. Most of us are completely unaware how our food is grown, the farming practices that went into that food and the health of the animals that we are consuming. Food manufacturers rely on our ignorance to sell their products. But no longer are we blindly purchasing these items. Consumers are demanding healthier, sustainable and organic foods. Cindy shows you how to make informed choices and save time and money while doing so.

Cindy's book is putting the knowledge in your hands. Pick it up!

—Dr. Josh Axe, DC, CNS

Introduction

My Journey to Wellness

I was raised in Middle America in the 1970s and I ate the same foods as the rest of our suburban neighbors. I grew up eating canned soups, toaster pastries, oatmeal cream pies, school lunches, frozen dinners, fast food burgers, tacos, brightly colored popsicles and as much candy as I could shovel in my mouth. Of course, my mom cooked dinner most every night of the week, but she had grown accustomed to convenience items like canned vegetables, boxed stuffing mixes, and the cheapest cut of meat on sale at the grocery store.

When I moved away from home, my diet consisted of low-fat and fat-free everything, canned foods, anything I could pop in a microwave and high-sugar juices. The result? By age 25, I was diagnosed with Hashimoto's Thyroiditis (an autoimmune thyroid disease). I didn't give my diagnosis a second thought. I took my prescribed medication and assumed that feeling tired, cold and headachy was my new way of life. I also suffered from frequent migraines, chronic bronchitis and low energy. I wasn't overweight, though. Not yet, anyway.

I was always interested in fitness and even majored in Physical Education and Health in college. I danced, exercised regularly and worked as a personal trainer. But I was following the USDA guidelines for nutrition. Remember the pyramid? I was told fat was bad and that I should eat 6 to 11 servings of bread, cereal and pasta a day...which I did. Do you think I eventually became overweight? You betcha!

Years later, after having two children, I became very tired all the time, had horrible allergies, frequent colds, sinus infections and bronchitis as well as frequent migraines, wicked PMS and high cholesterol. I was also about forty-five pounds overweight and was falling apart by the time I hit forty years old!

I wanted to exercise. I wanted to feel better, but I wasn't sure where to start and had no energy to do anything. I thought I was eating healthy by avoiding all fat and soda. I was eating fat-free cookies, fat-free mayo, "healthy" frozen meals and keeping an eye out for "natural" products. I even avoided nuts and avocadoes because of their high-fat content! When it came to food shopping, I never really thought about reading food labels. I grabbed the cheapest item on the shelf. I did occasionally look at the fat grams and sometimes the calorie count, but it never crossed my mind that the chemicals in my food were making me sick and overweight.

In 2009, I met an Integrative Nutrition Health Coach. She taught me some amazing things about our food supply today and how I could improve my health by not eating processed foods and conventionally farmed meats and dairy. She helped me listen to my body and determine if certain foods were causing my myriad symptoms. I slowly started educating myself and began reading ingredient labels. Since September 2010, I have been eating whole foods, farm-fresh eggs, and grass-fed meats. I eliminated dairy, soy and gluten, and I now grow a lot of my own food. I also incorporated daily exercise. I didn't join a gym. I simply started working out in my basement with weights and a used stationary bike. The result? I lost 50 pounds, had no more migraines or allergies, and my thyroid condition was under control. I'm now off all medications and haven't had a sinus infection or bronchitis since I stopped dairy. In addition, my cholesterol is normal and I have tons of energy all day long for my active kids!

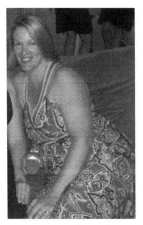

Before, 2010

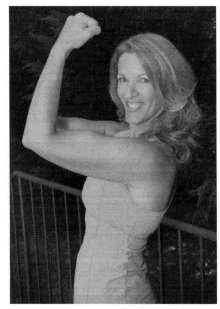

After, 2012

I even managed to get my husband and kids on board and they don't drink juice anymore. We've nixed the frozen chicken nuggets and fish sticks, and they now enjoy the same dinner as the adults. It is possible to get your kids to love broccoli, zucchini and kale—it just takes some time and creativity!

In 2012, I enrolled in the world's largest nutrition school, the Institute for Integrative Nutrition®, where I was trained in more than one hundred dietary theories. I studied a variety of practical lifestyle coaching methods. I was eager to share my new-found knowledge with the world and let people know that you don't have to feel this ill. You don't have to grow old and become sick and take lots of medication. I'm excited to share with others the amazing, life-changing experience I went through.

Today, I see so many clients with diet-related diseases and it makes me mad that our food supply has become so tainted with chemicals, hormones, pesticides and genetically-modified organisms. It's not your fault. I also have many family members who have developed chronic diseases who then go on to make changes to their diet and lifestyle, but what if you could avoid the cost and heartache associated with diet-related diseases in the first place?

My wish is for you to be inspired to take responsibility for your health now, no matter your age or state of health. No change is too small! Reading this book is an important step toward improving your health. So many of my friends and clients have improved their health, lost weight and weaned themselves off medications after making these simple changes. It may seem like a daunting task to overhaul your family's lifestyle and eating habits, so I'm hoping to make that easier for you in this step-by-step guide toward going unprocessed.

Please understand that this is a guide to educate you about the state of our food and help you learn how to prepare simple, healthy meals for your family. There will certainly be times when a quick, fast-food meal may be your only option and you'll just have to be OK with that and know that this isn't a lifestyle that requires 100 percent compliance. I don't want you to add stress to your life by creating restrictions and no-no lists. You'll slip. I slip too. We are all human, but as long as you can apply this lifestyle to 80 to 90 percent of the foods you eat, you can achieve better health and perhaps even lose weight!

You can do this!

Cindy

When you change a belief, you change everything.
~ Tony Robbins

How to use this book

I've outlined three steps to take you through your new food journey. In Step One, you'll learn how to decipher food labels and learn what to look for when shopping for food. We will build upon this new-found knowledge by swapping out some of your current staples with healthier versions in Step Two. Some regular items may become occasional treats or maybe you'll even develop distaste for them. I was amazed at how my appetite changed and my usual go-to items now had a chemical taste to them or were too sweet for my newly cleansed palate.

The third step is to create your healthy shopping lists and family meal plans. I'll show you how to save on healthy food, where to find it when you travel and how to get your family members on board. Then, we'll go in the kitchen and whip up some healthy meals in as little as ten minutes! I'm not recommending a specific diet like Paleo, Low-Carb or Vegetarian. I'm advocating for clean, whole and unprocessed foods. You can adapt the recipes if you need gluten, dairy or nut-free recipes. Slowly changing your habits over time can lead to success over a lifetime.

Step One:
Education and Awareness

Chapter 1: What is Processed Food?

Our food today comes in some pretty amusing shapes. We've got yogurt in tubes, butter in tubs, biscuits in cans, protein in a powder, and 100-calorie packs of chemically-processed food-like products. Chips come in every shape, size and color and there are over 300 different types of breakfast cereal to choose from!

For most American families, processed and packaged foods make up 75 percent of their diet. We've got frozen waffles, toaster pastries and sugar-coated cereals for breakfast; highly processed bread with nitrate-laden meats for lunch; and dinner can even come in a bag that you reheat on the stove in five minutes!

You probably grew up eating a certain way. Maybe your family only ate home-cooked meals. Maybe you lived on a farm. Or maybe you lived in the city and dined out for almost every meal. We learn our food habits when we are young, and these habits stick with us as we grow up and start our own families. Your family's diet is passed on from generation to generation—unless you break that tradition.

But how did we get here? Packaged and processed foods allow us the convenience of eating on the run, swinging through the drive-through or plopping a microwave dinner on the table in 2 minutes and 30 seconds. Why are our lives so rushed that we can't even take 20 minutes to prepare a fresh meal made with whole ingredients? We have put our health on the back burner in the name of convenience.

Shopping for healthy food has become difficult as well. Organic foods can be more expensive. Grass-fed meat can be hard to find. Marketing claims on the front of food packaging often misleads us into choosing something that is downright unhealthy. Have you ever noticed how many feet are devoted to processed food in the grocery store? Each aisle is on average 80 feet long, consisting of products such as soda, bread and cereal as well as chips, canned food and condiments. That's 480 feet of processed and packaged non-nutritious food. Food manufacturers are also getting savvy at creating concoctions of food that are engineered to flood the brain with dopamine and turn us into addicts.[1] Studies have found similarities between processed food and drugs of abuse, like heroin and cocaine.[2] It's the main reason why some people just can't stop eating these foods, no matter how hard they try. Their brain biochemistry has been hacked by the dopamine release that occurs in the brain when certain foods are consumed.[3]

Most of that processed food contains two common ingredients: white flour and white sugar. White flour is denatured, hybridized wheat with added gluten. The sugar is highly refined and could possibly be made from genetically modified sugar beets and causes numerous health problems when consumed in excess. I'm going to show you how to spot these overly processed ingredients and swap them for healthier alternatives.

Why should we ditch the processed food?

In a typical day at a local doctor's office, you'll find numerous patients being seen for endocrine disorders, respiratory infections and high blood pressure. They also come in with migraines, irritable bowel syndrome, complications due to diabetes and so on. Most of these health issues are diet-related. The growing number of people with obesity, diabetes and heart disease in America is caused by a non-nutritious diet and poor lifestyle management techniques.

Our current medical community focuses on our symptoms and not the root cause of a particular health issue. This model is how we've become a prescription-dependent society. Prescribing healthy food would be a much more effective medicine.

Consider these facts:

Seventy percent of Americans and nearly 1.5 billion people world-wide are overweight. More people will die today from the effects of obesity than ever before. During the past 20 years, there has been a dramatic increase in obesity in the United States and rates remain high. More than one-third of U.S. adults (34.9 percent) and approximately 17 percent (or 12.7 million) of children and adolescents aged 2 to 19 years are obese.

Two out of three adults and one out of three children in the United States are overweight or obese,[4,5] and the nation spends an estimated $190 billion a year treating obesity-related health conditions.

As noted in a 2014 article by investigative health reporter Martha Rosenberg,[6] the weight of the average American increased by 24 pounds in the four decades between 1960 and 2000.

According to Euromonitor, the average US citizen consumes more than 126 grams of sugar per day, more than any other country in the world.

About 600,000 people die of heart disease in the United States every year–that's one in every four deaths.

Heart disease is the leading cause of death for both men and women. Men made up more than half of the deaths due to heart disease in 2009.[7,8]

According to the CDC, more than 21 million Americans had diabetes in 2011. In 2010, there were 57,638 adolescents diagnosed with Type 2 Diabetes. In 1980, there were no new cases.

We've been eating eggs, meat and butter for hundreds of years, yet mainstream media and some doctors will demonize them. Heart disease, obesity and diabetes have just gained epidemic status in the last 20–30 years. It makes better sense to look at the amount of processed food with added sugar, refined grains, chemical preservatives and vegetable oils that have been added to our food over the last few decades.

You may ask, "Why should I worry about a specific chemical in my food or one ingredient in particular?" It's a matter of the dosage. There are certain ingredients like high-fructose corn syrup and soybean oil that are in 75 percent of processed foods. High-fructose corn syrup is in every ketchup bottle on almost every restaurant table in the U.S. It's in salad dressings, mayo, bread, soda and hundreds of other foods. Almost every restaurant in the country uses vegetable oil that is comprised of 100 percent soybean oil, corn oil or canola (all GMO and inflammatory) in their cooking methods and marinades. It's nearly impossible to avoid soy. Artificial colors are another chemical ingredient prevalent in our food today. Most of the ingredients on the FDA's Generally Recognized as Safe (GRAS) list have been there for almost 50 years and nearly all of them are untested for their safety. The FDA admits that they don't have the resources to test our food. They leave that up to the manufacturers.

Another untested area of our food is Genetically Modified Organisms. We need to discuss GMOs first because they are in roughly 80 percent of processed foods.[9]

What are Genetically Modified Organisms?

A GMO (genetically modified organism) is the result of a laboratory process where genes from the DNA of one species are extracted and artificially forced into the genes of an unrelated plant or animal. The foreign genes may come from bacteria, viruses, insects, animals or even humans. Because this involves the transfer of genes, GMOs are also known as "transgenic" organisms. This process may be called either Genetic Engineering (GE) or Genetic Modification (GM); they are one and the same.

There are eight GM food crops. The five major varieties—soy, corn, canola, cotton, and sugar beets—have bacterial genes inserted, which allow the plants to survive an otherwise deadly dose of weed killer. Farmers use considerably more herbicides on these GM crops, so the food has higher herbicide residues. About 68 percent of GM crops are herbicide-tolerant.

The second GM trait is a built-in pesticide found in GM corn and cotton. A gene from the soil bacterium called Bt (for Bacillus thuringiensis) is inserted into the plant's DNA, where it secretes the insect-killing Bt-toxin in every cell. About 19 percent of GM crops produce their own pesticide. Another 13 percent produce a pesticide and are herbicide-tolerant.

One alarming aspect of the whole GMO debate is the fact that so many Americans are going about their daily lives completely unaware that they are consuming genetically modified organisms at just about every meal. The reason I know this is because I used to be completely unaware of them.

Here are the current GMO crops in the United States:

- 95% of sugar beet crops are GMO
- 94% of soy crops are GMO
- 88% of corn crops are GMO
- 90% of rapeseed (canola) crops are GMO
- 90% of cotton (cottonseed oil) crops are GMO (foods and livestock feed)

In addition:
- More than 50% of Hawaiian papaya crops are GMO
- Over 24,000 acres of zucchini and yellow squash are GMO
- GMO Arctic Golden and Arctic Granny apples, which were

approved in February 2015, may hit store shelves in 2016.

- Products derived from the above crops are also made of GMOs, including oils from all seed crops, soy protein, soy lecithin, aspartame, cornstarch, corn syrup and high-fructose corn syrup among others.

Why should we be concerned about them?

The term "genetic modification" is used both commonly and legally to refer to the use of recombinant DNA techniques, in ways that are not possible or desirable in nature, to transfer genetic material between organisms. This concept of genetic modification brings about alterations in genetic makeup and in the properties of the organism developed. This technique is highly mutagenic and leads to unpredictable changes in the DNA and proteins produced by the GMO that can lead to toxic or allergic reactions.

GM proponents will argue that "genetic modification" has been used for centuries in an attempt to blur the lines and create confusion. Traditional genetics used selective breeding, tissue cultures, hybridization and other methods that assist nature but does not circumvent natural laws.

The methods used to transfer the genes of modified DNA of a genetically modified plant are imprecise and unpredictable. These unintended changes are possible differences in the food's nutritional values, toxic and allergic effects, lower crop yields and unforeseen harm to the environment.

Crops such as Bt cotton produce pesticides inside the plant. This kills or deters insects, saving the farmer from having to spray pesticides. The plants themselves are toxic—and not just to insects. Farmers in India, who let their sheep graze on Bt cotton plants after the harvest, saw thousands of sheep die![10]

Why should we be extremely wary of consuming any food that has been genetically altered? Here are five reasons why:

1. **GMOs are unhealthy.** Since the introduction of GMOs in the mid-1990s, the number of food allergies has sky-rocketed, and health issues such as autism, digestive problems and reproductive disorders are on the rise. Animal testing with GMOs has resulted in cases of organ failure, digestive disorders, infertility and accelerated aging. Despite an announcement in 2012 by the American Medical Association stating they saw no reason for labeling genetically modified foods, the American Academy of Environmental Medicine has urged doctors to prescribe non-GMO diets for their patients.

2. **They increase herbicide use.** When chemical giant, Monsanto, came up with the idea for Round-up Ready crops, the theory was to make the crops resistant to the pesticide that would normally kill them. This meant the farmers could spray the crops, killing the surrounding weeds and pests without doing any harm to the crops themselves. However, after a number of years have passed, many weeds and pests have themselves become resistant to the spray, and herbicide-use increased (both in amount and strength) by 11 percent between 1996 and 2011. This translates to lots more pesticide residue in our foods. Yum!

3. **They are everywhere!** GMOs make up about 70 to 80 percent of our foods in the United States. Most foods that contain GMOs are processed foods. But they also exist in the form of fresh vegetables such as corn on the cob, papaya and squash. The prize for the top two most genetically modified crops in the United States goes to corn and soy. Think about

how many foods in your pantry or refrigerator contain corn or its byproducts (high-fructose corn syrup) or soy and its byproducts (partially hydrogenated soybean oil).

4. **GM crops don't ensure larger harvests.** As it turns out, GMO crop yields are not as promising as some projections implied. In fact, in some instances, they have been out-yielded by their non-GMO counterparts. This conclusion was reached in a 20-year study carried out by the University of Wisconsin and funded by the U.S. Department of Agriculture, thus negating one of the main arguments in favor of GMOs.

5. **U.S. labeling suppression.** Many of the companies who have an interest in keeping GMOs on the market don't want you to know which foods contain them. For this reason, they have suppressed recent attempts by states such as California, Washington and Colorado to require labeling of GMO products. And since these companies have deep pockets, they were successful—for now. The companies who spent the most on these campaigns are Monsanto (who produces the GMO seeds), Pepsi, Coca Cola, Nestle and General Mills, which produce some of the most processed foods in existence. Incidentally, most other developed countries, such as the nations of the European Union, Japan, Australia, Brazil and China have mandatory labeling of genetically modified foods.

In 2009, the American Academy of Environmental Medicine (AAEM) stated that, "Several animal studies indicate serious health risks associated with genetically modified (GM) food," including infertility, immune problems, accelerated aging, faulty insulin regulation and changes in major organs and the gastrointestinal system. The AAEM has asked physicians to advise all patients to avoid GM foods.[11,12]

Between 1996 and 2008, US farmers sprayed an extra 383 million pounds of herbicide on GMOs. Overuse of Roundup results in "super-weeds" resistant to the herbicide. This is causing farmers to use even more toxic herbicides every year. Not only does this create environmental harm, GM foods contain higher residues of toxic herbicides. Roundup, for example, is linked with sterility, hormone disruption, birth defects and cancer. A skin prick allergy test shows that some people react to GM soy but not to wild, natural soy.[13]

Bt Corn and GM Cotton linked to allergies

The biotech industry claims that Bt-toxin is harmless to humans and mammals because the natural bacteria version has been used as a spray by farmers for years. In reality, hundreds of people exposed to Bt spray had allergic-type symptoms,[14] and mice fed Bt had powerful immune responses[15] and damaged intestines.[16] Moreover, the Bt in GM crops is designed to be more toxic than the natural spray and is thousands of times more concentrated.

How do I avoid GMOs?

GMOs are not currently labeled in the US. There are 64 countries around the globe that do require GMO labeling. If you don't wish to partake of GMO foods, what can you do? First and foremost, buy organic. The USDA has strict guidelines for producers of organic foods, which restrict them from using any GMO products in their foods.[17]

If a food is not organically grown, look for a Non-GMO Project Seal, which certifies that it has been tested and found to have less than 0.9 percent GMO-contamination.

The Argument for Grass-fed and Pastured Meat

One of the last changes I made to our family's diet was to incorporate grass-fed meat from local farmers. It was last because it truly is more expensive and, to be honest, it took me a while to wrap my head around the concept of paying double or triple per pound for certain cuts of meat. However, I noticed that I felt better and had better digestion when I consumed grass-fed meat.

Also, when given proper nutrition, such as grazing on high-quality pasture, cattle produce less methane gas, a potent greenhouse gas. Grass-fed meats contain higher levels of omega-3 fatty acids.[18] Grass-fed beef contains between 2 and 5 times more omega-3s than grain-fed beef. Beef is one of the best dietary sources of conjugated linoleic acid (CLA), and grass-fed beef contains an average of 2 to 3 times more CLA than grain-fed beef. Research has shown that CLA might be protective against heart disease, diabetes and cancer.[19]

Plus, after seeing videos and pictures from conventionally raised meats, I couldn't support that kind of industry any longer. Cattle and chicken farmers market their meat with pictures of happy cows and chickens tromping through grassy fields. This is far from the reality of the confined animal feeding operation or CAFO. This is what the meat industry counts on—your blind ignorance.

The Union of Concerned Scientists has this to say about CAFO meats:

1. At least 70 percent of all large cattle feedlots incorporate antibiotics into daily feed. The ratio is 0.25 pounds of antibiotic per 15 to 20 lbs of feed. At least one-fourth of smaller feedlots use antibiotics in the same way.

2. In the pork industry, 90 percent of all starter feeds and 75 percent of all grower feeds contain antibiotics.

3. The Union of Concerned Scientists (UCSUSA.org) has

estimated that a total of 24.6 million total pounds of antibiotics were used for non-medical purposes in US meat production, including 10.3 million pounds in hogs, 10.5 million pounds in chickens and 3.7 million pounds in cattle.

4. Most ranchers/farmers allow a drug withdrawal period before slaughter in order to reduce drug levels in the edible tissues. However, even after a 2-week period, antibiotic levels may still be high enough that a penicillin or sulfa-sensitive person may have an allergic reaction to the drug residue in meats.

Still can't afford grass-fed meat? Try pork or chicken. The U.S. Department of Agriculture (USDA) does not allow the use of hormones in pigs, chickens, turkeys and other fowl. That is why you'll see the term "no hormones added" on labels of pork or poultry products along with the statement, "Federal regulations prohibit the use of hormones."

You'll find some resources to find grass-fed and pastured meats in the Resources section in the back of this book.

Do I really need to buy organic dairy?

Short answer: absolutely! If you can tolerate dairy, and not too many people can, it should be organic and raw if you can find it. Conventional dairy products have high amounts of hormones, pesticides, GMO feed and antibiotics. Any dairy, whether organic or conventional, contains a high level of hormones because the milk is intended to help calves grow. It contains natural growth hormones, such as IGF-1, an insulin-like growth factor. Those same growth hormones can cause weight gain and acne for you.

Some dairy farmers give their cows rBGH, recombinant bovine growth hormone, a genetically modified hormone that forces a cow to give more milk than nature intended. Feeding cows corn instead of their natural diet of grass causes acidosis, an acid overload that leads to ulcers and bleeding in the stomach. For this, the cows are given antibiotics, which we consume as well.

About 75 percent of the worldwide population is lactose-intolerant; they lack the enzymes needed to digest the lactose found in dairy. Symptoms can include gas, bloating, diarrhea, eczema, coughing, post-nasal drip and congestion. Pasteurized milk is heated to such high temperatures that it kills the enzyme, lactase, which is necessary to digest the milk sugar, lactose. High-heat pasteurization also kills the good bacteria or probiotics along with vitamins and other enzymes.

Grass-fed cows' milk is higher in conjugated linoleic acid, beta-carotene, essential fatty acids and vitamins A and E. Still, it is best if you can find raw, grass-fed milk from a local farmer, because organic milk at the grocery store is going to be heated at high temperatures, killing the beneficial nutrients.

The Nasty 9

The following ingredients are what I call the **Nasty 9**. This is what you should strive to stay away from when purchasing your food. Unfortunately, this is not a complete list of the hundreds of chemicals found in our food, but these are the major ones that can cause the most harm because they are found in the majority of processed foods. Most of the time if you avoid these ingredients in a particular food, you'll find it won't contain too many other unmentionables. I don't like to label food as good or bad; instead, I separate it into nutritious or non-nutritious. If your food contains these ingredients, you can bet it's non-nutritious.

1. **High-Fructose Corn Syrup (HFCS)**

   What is it? HFCS is made from GMO corn (a government-subsidized crop). The corn is steeped, milled and broken down into 55 percent fructose and 45 percent glucose. There are even some forms of HFCS that are 90 percent fructose. It became a popular sweetener in the late 1970s when the price of regular sugar was high, while corn prices were low due to government subsidies.

   Why should I avoid it? Fructose is metabolized by the liver. When you consume too much, it gets converted into fat.[20] HFCS raises triglyceride levels and contributes to an increase in body weight and body fat.[21] It's also linked to non-alcohol fatty liver disease[22] and has detrimental effects on metabolism.[23, 24]

2. **Partially Hydrogenated Oils**

   What is it? Partially hydrogenated oils (PHOs), or artificial trans fats, are created when you add hydrogen molecules into vegetable oils which, in turn, changes the chemical structure of the oils from a liquid to a solid. PHOs have been used since the 1950s to increase the shelf life and flavor stability of processed foods.[25]

   Why should I avoid it? Clinical trials and observational studies both indicate that trans fats increase inflammation, especially in people who are overweight or obese. Inflammation in the body can lead to heart disease, diabetes, obesity and numerous other health issues. PHOs also increase LDL (Low Density Lipoproteins), otherwise known as the "bad" cholesterol. Even the FDA now states that trans fats are unhealthy and have been linked to coronary heart disease. In

1999, they asked manufacturers to eliminate the ingredient; however, you can still find PHOs in crackers, frosting, snack foods, popcorn, shortening, coffee creamers, frozen goods, cakes and refrigerated biscuits and rolls.[26, 27]

Interesting Note: A misleading labeling loophole allows food manufacturers to claim "0 grams trans fats" if their product has less than 0.5 grams of trans fats per serving. But if partially hydrogenated oils are listed on the ingredient label and you consume more than the recommended serving, you're consuming an unknown amount of trans fats.

3. **MSG or Monosodium Glutamate**
   Alternative names: yeast extract, hydrolyzed vegetable protein, autolyzed yeast and many products with isolates, such as soy protein isolates.

   What is it? MSG is a flavor enhancer that literally excites your brain cells to death. It is the sodium salt of the amino acid glutamic acid. It is made commercially by the fermentation of molasses but exists in many products made from fermented proteins, such as soy sauce and hydrolyzed vegetable protein.

   Why should I avoid it? MSG can create serious bodily reactions like headache, dizziness, tingling muscles, fast heart rate, anxiety and chest tightness. People with asthma may find that glutamates complicate or worsen their symptoms.[28] A study published in 2008 in the *Journal Obesity* indicated that MSG intake may be associated with increased risk of being overweight.

4. **Artificial Sweeteners**

   Alternative names: Aspartame (Equal, Nutra-Sweet), Sucralose (Splenda), Acesulfame Potassium (K), Saccharin (Sweet'N Low), bleached white Stevia (Truvia), Neotame

   What is it? Artificial sugars are sugar substitutes used to sweeten diet soft drinks, gum, mints, sugar-free foods and beverages.

   Why should I avoid it? The Center for Science in the Public Interest (CSPI) cautions everyone to avoid **aspartame**, **saccharin** and **acesulfame K** because they are unsafe consumed in large amounts or are very poorly tested and not worth the risk. Numerous studies performed on laboratory rats link aspartame and saccharin to cancer, including a seven-year study conducted by a major nonprofit oncology lab in Italy.[29]

   The FDA is hesitant to reply to these concerns because "putting restrictions on aspartame would come at a significant cost. Food companies and consumers around the world bought about $570 million worth of it in 2005. New regulatory action on aspartame would also jeopardize the *billions* of dollars worth of products sold with it."[30]

   Aspartame is of particular concern because it contains phenylalanine (50%), aspartic acid (40%) and methanol (10%), three well-recognized neurotoxins. It's also a GMO. The following symptoms have been associated with the consumption of aspartame.

headaches	nausea	dizziness
hearing loss	tinnitus	insomnia
blurred vision	eye problems	hallucinations
memory loss	slurred speech	mild to suicidal depression
personality changes	violent episodes	mood changes
anxiety attacks	hyperactivity	heart arrhythmia
edema or swelling	gastrointestinal disorders	seizures
skin lesions	muscle cramps	joint pains
fatigue	PMS	menstrual irregularities
chest pain	increased appetite	numbness and tingling of extremities

Fortunately, most of the above symptoms are alleviated once aspartame use is discontinued.

5. **Refined Sugar**

   What is it? Ninety-five percent of US sugar crops are GMO sugar beets. The process of refining involves different stages of washing, simmering, centrifuging, filtering and, finally, drying. The last stage involves using bleaching agents such as carbon dioxide or lime to whiten the sugar. It involves the introduction of limewater (milk of lime, or calcium hydroxide suspension) and carbon dioxide enriched gas into the "raw juice" (the sugar-rich liquid prepared from the diffusion stage of the process) to form calcium carbonate and precipitate impurities that are then removed.

   Why should I avoid it? Besides the obvious effects like dental cavities and an increase in calories, sugar is pervasive in the American diet and causes myriad health effects. Sugar can feed cancer cells,[31] promote insulin resistance, decrease the amount of leptin hormone (which controls appetite) and cause weight gain. Also, products containing sugar as an ingredient may very well be from GMO Sugar Beets, but we can't be completely sure because GMO's are not (currently) labeled in the U.S.

6. **Abbreviated additives** such as:

BHA. Butylated Hydroxyanisole A is a petroleum-derived preservative that helps prevent spoilage due to oxidation. The US National Institutes of Health states that BHA is "reasonably anticipated to be a human carcinogen based on evidence of carcinogenicity in experimental animals." Banned in Japan. Found in cereals, baked goods, instant foods and ice cream. Known to cause allergic reactions and neuro-toxic effects, including hyperactivity.

BHT. Butylated Hydroxytoluene is added to most foods to preserve fats and slow down the oxidation rate that can change taste or color. It is primarily made from the chemicals p-Cresol & isobutylene. P-Cresol is a chemical that is a mosquito attractant while isobutylene is a flammable substance one hydrocarbon away from common butane. Produces hyperactivity in children.

TBHQ. Tertiary Butylhydroquinone is a form of butane linked to cancer and DNA damage in lab animals. This chemical is made from butane (a toxic gas) and can only be used at a rate of 0.02 percent of the total oil in a product. Consuming as little as one gram of this chemical has been shown to cause health issues like ADHD in children, to asthma, allergies and dermatitis in adults. It has even been known to cause stomach cancer in laboratory animals.

Calcium Disodium EDTA. It is made from formaldehyde, sodium cayanide and Ethylenediamine. Calcium Disodium is often used as a drug to stop lead poisoning or to treat someone exposed to radioactivity. It causes your body to expel heavy metals.

BVO. Brominated Vegetable Oil or BVO is derived from soybean oil with bromine added. Bromine is a fire retardant and can be found in sports drinks and some sodas. It helps prevent the citrus oils from rising to the surface. It also ensures the stability of the flavor mixture. It can accumulate in fatty tissue and cause organ damage.

ADA. Azodicarbonamide is a dough conditioner used mostly in breads in fast food restaurants and beyond. It's banned in Europe and Australia and if you're caught using it in Singapore, you're headed to jail for 15 years! During bread making, ADA breaks down into chemicals that can cause tumors in mice as well as respiratory issues, allergies and asthma in humans.[32]

7. **Nitrates, Nitrites**

   What are they? Sodium Nitrates and Potassium Nitrites help preserve food, inhibit the growth of bacteria and give bacon, hot dogs, salami and other packaged and cured meats their signature pink color. They're also found in drinking water thanks to nitrogen-based fertilizers as well as livestock waste. Nitrates occur in vegetables such as celery and spinach, but do not pose a health threat in their natural state.

   Why should I avoid them? When nitrates are heated, they can combine with certain amino acids to create carcinogenic nitrosamines. These carcinogens can cause an array of cancers in both children and adults. One study, published in the March 1994 issue of "Cancer Causes and Control," shows a correlation between childhood brain tumors and eating cured meats once or twice a week.[33] Researchers also found that women who consumed hot dogs more than once a week while pregnant were more likely to have children with brain tumors. They have been linked to diseases like leukemia and non-Hodgkin lymphoma as well as ovarian, colon, rectal, bladder, stomach, esophageal, pancreatic and thyroid cancer.

8. **Carrageenan**

   What is it? Carrageenan is a food additive extracted from red seaweed. It's used as an emulsifier and thickener in processed foods like non-dairy milks, ice cream, infant formula and yogurt.

   Why should I avoid it? Ingestion can cause inflammation that leads to gastrointestinal cancers, ulcerations and inflammatory bowel. Even low doses can cause glucose intolerance and impaired insulin action, both of which are precursors to diabetes.[34]

9. **Artificial Colors** (Red #40, Blue #6, Yellow #5, etc . . .)

   What are they? Food dyes are derived from both coal tar and petroleum and can be found in many foods. Companies like using them because they are cheaper, stabler and brighter than most natural colorings. However, consumers are moving toward the more natural approaches and companies are beginning to eliminate food colorings or switch to safer natural food colorings such as beta carotene, paprika, beet juice and turmeric.

   Why should I avoid them? Artificial colors are derived

from Aniline, a toxic, volatile petroleum compound, that is toxic by inhalation of the vapor, ingestion or percutaneous absorption.

Many dyes have been banned in other countries because of their adverse effects on laboratory animals.

Research on these approved dyes below demonstrated the following effects:

Blue 1 Used in baked goods, beverages, dessert powders, candies, cereals, drugs and other products. This dye caused tumors and hypersensitivity reactions in mice.

Blue 2 Used in colored beverages, candies, pet foods and many other foods and drugs. This dye caused brain tumors in male rats.

Citrus Red 2 Permitted only for coloring the skin of oranges. This particular dye caused tumors of the urinary bladder and other organs in rodents.

Green 3 Used in candies, beverages, dessert powders, ice cream, sorbet and other foods. This dye caused bladder and testes tumors in male rats.

Orange B Used in sausage casings. Testing did not reveal any problems.

Red 3 Used in maraschino cherries, sausage casings, oral drugs, baked goods and candies. This dye caused thyroid cancer in animals. This dye is banned in cosmetics and externally applied drugs. However, the FDA still allows Red 3 in ingested drugs and food.

Red 40 Used in beverages, bakery goods, dessert powders, candies, cereals, food, drugs and cosmetics. This dye caused immune system tumors and hypersensitivity in mice. It may also trigger hyperactivity in children.

Yellow 5 Used in bakery goods, beverages, dessert powders, candies, cereals, gelatin desserts, pet foods and cosmetics. This dye may be contaminated with several cancer-causing chemicals. It caused hypersensitivity reactions. It may also trigger hyperactivity and behavioral effects in children.

Yellow 6 Used in bakery goods, cereals, beverages, dessert powders, candies, gelatin desserts, sausage, cosmetics, drugs and other foods. This dye caused adrenal tumors and occasionally caused severe hypersensitivity reactions.

These food dyes cannot be considered safe. However, the FDA has yet to ban them.

The Nasty 9

- High-Fructose Corn Syrup
- Partially Hydrogenated Oils
- Aspartame, Sucralose, Acesulfame K, Neotame
- MSG
- Refined Sugar
- BHA, BHT, BVO, EDTA, TBHQ, ADA
- Sodium Nitrates, Nitrites
- Carrageenan
- Artificial Colors

HEALTH COACH TIP

Take a picture of the Nasty 9 and take it with you when you go shopping.

Chapter 2: Becoming a Label Detective

Cheap, processed food is available everywhere, not just the grocery store. You'll find it in school cafeterias, the office supply store, airplanes, gas stations, even foreign countries that allow U.S. food manufacturers to sell there. They make it very easy for us to have non-nutritious food at every corner.

Unfortunately, this highly processed food is damaging our health to a great degree. We have to learn how to become food sleuths and decipher what is going on inside the box. We have to learn how to read food ingredient labels in order to avoid eating added chemicals, GMOs, pesticides and preservatives. When you come across an ingredient you're not sure about, you can use **BeFoodSmart.com** to research a particular item in their vast database. They will give the ingredient a grade and list the health effects associated with any given item.

HEALTH COACH TIP

Set an intention to eliminate a few non-nutritious foods from your diet. Share that intention with others on social media or with a friend. Having support is key in creating and changing lifestyle habits.

Food Marketing and Labeling Claims

Even I have been fooled by a snazzy marketing claim on the front of a food package. Food manufacturers have designed packaging to draw us in and capture us within a few seconds with bold claims and bright colors. But the truth lies in the Ingredient Label, and even then, sometimes it still isn't clear what our food is made from.

Here are some of the attention-grabbing claims and catchphrases we frequently see on food containers:

Natural

Has no legal meaning. A certain bread manufacturer used to claim this on their label, but used Azodicarbonamide (a dangerous dough conditioner) in their bread.

Enriched

Describes the process of adding back in at least some of the nutrients lost during processing with synthetic vitamins that our bodies usually don't absorb or recognize.

All-Natural Meat & Dairy Products

The USDA states a "natural" animal product as one that does not contain additives, preservatives or colors. This label does not tell us if the animals were given antibiotics, hormones or what they were fed.

Whole Grain claims

Grain products should list fiber on the Nutrition Facts as proof that they are made from the whole grain. Look for products with two or more grams of fiber in every one hundred calories. If it contains one gram or less of fiber, then it's a whole grain imposter! Refined grains have the germ and bran removed, which is the nutritious part of a whole grain, leaving you with the starchy endosperm. This is why refined grains are required to be enriched—their nutrients are lost.

0 Grams Trans fat

As I stated in the Nasty 9, a misleading labeling loophole allows food manufacturers to claim "0 Grams Trans fats" if their product has less than 0.5 grams of trans fats per serving. But, if partially hydrogenated oils are listed on the ingredient label, you are consuming unknown amounts of trans fats!

Special logos from organizations

Some packaged foods, like cereal and snack food, carry big fancy logos and check marks from organizations like the American Heart Association. These logos don't carry any weight at all and won't tell you if a food is highly processed with refined sugars, flours or even GMOs.

Organic

Foods labeled as organic must contain at least 95 percent organic ingredients. This is a better indicator than the "natural" label, because that one doesn't mean anything. The USDA Organic label on these products makes them easy to spot and ensures that the ingredients have met the USDA standards for organic certification.

Certified 100% Organic

This label, though hard to find, ensures that the food is both organically grown and does not contain any genetically modified organisms. This provides us with true transparency and is approved by the USDA for meeting the standards for this certification.

Non-GMO

Currently, there is no required testing or labeling for a manufacturer to make the claim that a product is non-GMO. However, a voluntary verification system is available that many companies choose to pay for so that you can be assured their product is not made with genetically modified ingredients. Look for the Project Non-GMO Verified label to ensure that the sources of the ingredients are verified and the product is not made with genetically modified organisms.

Gluten-free

You can make all sorts of food gluten free by using highly processed rice flours, potato starch and bean flours, but that doesn't make it the least bit healthy. You'll even find some of the Nasty 9 in GF foods. Don't forget to also read the ingredient label on these foods as well.

Cage-free Eggs

This means the poultry does not live inside cages, but they could still be kept indoors in warehouses with hundreds of thousands of other chickens. Vegetarian-fed chickens means they were likely fed GMO grains like corn and soy, which is not natural to a chicken's diet of grass and bugs. Free-range is better, which means the poultry were allowed to roam outdoors. The best option is pastured-raised, GMO-free eggs from a local farm.

DO THE FLIP!

I tell all my clients, friends and family to do this one thing to improve their health and that's FLIP over the box, jar or package and **READ THE LABEL**! We have to start reading those ingredient labels to understand what we are eating. Currently, GMOs are not

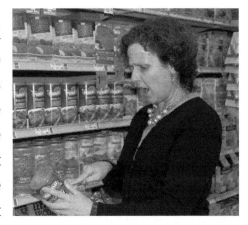

labeled in the US, but with some careful detective work, you can learn how to spot them.

Become a Sugar Detective. Sugar can be found in the most unusual places and under many aliases. You can bet it's a sugar if it ends in "-ose." You'll find about twenty different names for sugar on an ingredient label and some products will have multiple versions of it.

Beet sugar	Brown sugar	Lactose	Malt syrup	Rice syrup
Sucrose	Maltose	Fructose	Galactose	Corn syrup
Dextrose	Invert sugar	Evaporated cane juice	Glucose	Sorbitol
Mannitol	Xylitol	High-fructose corn syrup		

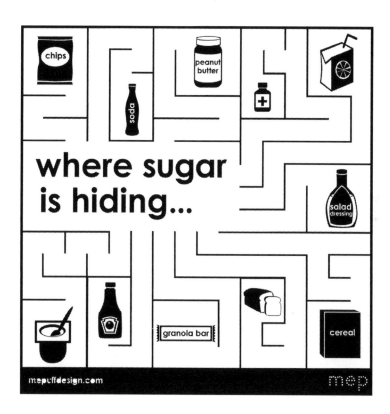

Step Two:
The Swaps

Chapter 3: Deconstructing the Food Label

When you look at an ingredient label, the first few ingredients are the basics of that food. Then you have preservatives to keep the item fresh; colorants that give the food a specific color; artificial flavors to deepen the existing flavor; texturants that either keep the item together or give it a particular texture; and stabilizers and thickeners that work with emulsifiers to keep fats and oils from separating. Additionally, you can have dough conditioners, whipping agents, gums, bleaching agents, moisture controllers and waxes. You'll find all of these in the simplest of foods, like grocery store bread.

I taught myself how to replicate certain tastes by looking at the whole food ingredients in a packaged food and weeding out the rest of the items. For example, take a look at the ingredients in this popular taco seasoning packet.

> <u>Salt</u>, Maltodextrin, <u>Chili Pepper</u>, <u>Red Pepper</u>, Monosodium Glutamate, Corn Starch, <u>Yellow Corn Flour</u>, <u>Spice</u>, <u>Sugar</u>. Contains less than 2% of: Citric Acid, Natural Flavor, Partially Hydrogenated Soybean Oil, Silicon Dioxide (Anticaking Agent), Yeast Extract, Ethoxyquin (Preservative)

The whole ingredients are underlined. Now you can't be really sure what the spices are, but it's for tacos and common spice profiles for Mexican food are cumin, garlic, chili powder, paprika, onion powder and salt. So, I came up with my own seasoning mix and stored it in a jar in my cupboards. (See recipe section.)

Now, let's do another one: "Cream of . . ." condensed soups

There are hundreds of these types of soups on the market, but as you'll see below, they're not healthy at all.

Chicken Stock, Wheat Flour, Chicken Fat, Chicken Meat Cooked, Cream, Corn Starch, Canola Oil, Corn Oil, Cottonseed Oil, Margarine, Chicken Mechanically Separated, Salt, Soybean Oil, Water, Beta Carotene, Calcium Caseinate, Flavors Chicken, Chicken Powder, Dairy Blend Dried, Whey Dried, Food Starch Modified, Monosodium Glutamate, Flavoring Natural, Sodium Phosphate, Soy Protein Concentrate, Soy Protein Isolate, Spices Extractive, Whey, Yeast Extract

There's not a lot of whole food here, but the basics are chicken stock, fat, flour and cream. Those are pretty much the ingredients you'll find in a "roux" or base for making sauces. I have a few recipes for making these sauces in the recipe section.

By learning how to adapt and deconstruct a recipe, you can pretty much transform any processed food into your own healthy creation!

How to Adapt Recipes

Recipe Calls For . . .	Healthy Alternatives	Considerations
flour	Use almond (NUT) flour/meal, gluten-free flour, unbleached flour, whole wheat flour.	Nut flours works for both savory and sweet recipes. They don't measure 1:1 though. You will need to adjust your wet ingredients.
cornstarch	Use arrowroot powder (a root plant, dehydrated at low temperature, then ground to create a binder to hold items together).	Arrowroot can be purchased in the whole food section at your grocery store. 2 tsp arrowroot = 1 tbsp cornstarch
Crisco	Use extra virgin unrefined coconut oil, lard or palm oil shortening.	Lard is the ideal healthy substitute for Crisco but since it's hard to come by, you can use coconut oil or palm shortening.

Recipe Calls For . . .	Healthy Alternatives	Considerations
milk	Use coconut milk (full-fat can); almond milk, raw cow's milk. *Avoid **Carrageenan**.	Other nut milks work well too! Try hazelnut milk or cashew milk for a different flavor profile. Rice milk is okay, but contains a lot of sugar.
flavored yogurt	Use plain coconut milk/almond milk yogurt, organic whole cow's milk and goat's milk.	Always buy plain yogurt and flavor it yourself with honey, cinnamon or fruit.
heavy cream	Use coconut milk.	Must be full-fat, canned coconut milk.
sugar	Use unfiltered raw honey, maple syrup grade B, coconut palm sugar (granulated), molasses, or Stevia.	Experiment by reducing the amount of sugar by 50%. For example, if a recipe calls for 1 cup of sugar, try using 1/2 cup honey/maple syrup/coconut sugar instead. You can always add more.
breadcrumbs	Use ground almonds mixed with some Himalayan sea salt and dried herbs (if desired).	Works with other nuts as well. Try pecans for a different flavor!
mayonnaise	Look for mayonnaise without soybean or canola oil. Buy full fat.	Use avocado instead. It's super creamy.
vegetable oil/canola oil	Use extra virgin unrefined organic coconut oil, organic extra virgin cold pressed olive oil, pasture-raised butter and ghee.	Use coconut oil or butter for temperatures above 250 degrees (sizzle).
soy sauce	Use tamari, coconut aminos.	Tamari is still a soy product but is gluten-free. Coconut aminos is a soy- and gluten-free product, which can be found in natural grocery stores or online.

Recipe Calls For . . .	Healthy Alternatives	Considerations
white flour pasta	Use steamed or sautéed vegetables or gluten-free brown rice pasta.	Try spiralized zucchini, yellow squash, carrots or sweet potato. Often what people crave about a pasta dish is the SAUCE, not the pasta noodles. Try making your favorite sauce and serve on steamed or sautéed veggies instead!
rice	Use cauliflower rice, wild rice, grains and seeds.	See Healthy Recipe Section.
mashed potatoes	Use real butter, 2% milk or stock with mashed cauliflower.	See Healthy Recipe Section.
wine	Use stock.	Use homemade vegetable, free range chicken, beef or fish stock.
cheese sauce	Use organic cheese melted with a splash of milk.	Use nut-based cream sauce; nutritional yeast (B12).
grated cheese	Omit or use nutritional yeast.	Grated cheese can very often just be eliminated from the recipe altogether.
peanut butter	Use almond butter, cashew butter, sun butter. Choose organic if you need peanut butter.	Use raw soaked nuts in sea salt for a few hours to make these nut butters.

Beyond the Basics

If you want to increase the nutrition in a given recipe, you can try upgrading your ingredients to these:

- Instead of cream . . . use full-fat canned coconut milk.
- Instead of wheat flour . . . use 3 parts almond flour, 1 part flax meal.

- Instead of vegetable oil . . . use coconut oil or ghee.
- Instead of sugar . . . use coconut sugar.
- Instead of corn syrup . . . use raw honey or real maple syrup.
- Instead of potatoes . . . use sweet potatoes.

Try making these changes by gradually swapping these highly processed foods for something healthier.

Processed Food	Swap For	Even Healthier
margarine	real butter	organic, or butter from grass-fed cows
skim milk	2% organic milk	raw milk or unsweetened almond milk, coconut milk
fruit-flavored yogurt	Plain yogurt with your own honey or fruit	raw milk or organic Greek yogurt
vegetable/canola oil	cold-pressed extra virgin olive oil, ghee	coconut oil, avocado oil, nut oils, ghee
roasted, salted nuts	unsalted nuts	raw, unsalted nuts
frozen fish sticks	pan-fried wild fish	grilled, baked, poached wild fish with herbs and spices
hamburger meat	hormone/antibiotic-free beef	grass-fed beef
frozen chicken (w/ added sodium solution)	chicken without added sodium	free-range, pastured organic chicken
canned vegetables	fresh or frozen veggies	organic, local fresh veggies
flavored coffee creamer	half & half	raw cream or milk
lunch meat	nitrate/nitrite-free meats	sliced turkey from the breast
fat-free mayonnaise	full-fat mayonnaise	homemade or organic mayonnaise
processed cheese slices	full-fat real cheese block	raw, organic, block of cheese
white flour	whole wheat flour	oat, spelt, gluten-free flours
white rice	brown rice	quinoa, millet, wild rice
regular enriched pasta	whole grain pasta	brown rice or quinoa pasta
table salt	Celtic sea salt	Himalayan and Celtic sea salts
sugar, artificial sugars	organic pure cane sugar	raw honey, Stevia, real maple syrup

Processed Food	Swap For	Even Healthier
soybean oil (in packaged foods), added soy	omit	omit
jar of parmesan cheese	fresh block parmesan	organic, hard cheese
jelly w/ high-fructose corn syrup	100% fruit jelly	homemade jam, preserves
soda, diet drinks, juice	sparkling water, flavored	plain filtered water with lemon
packaged mac 'n cheese	pasta with homemade cheese sauce	whole wheat pasta, with tomato sauce, herbs
condensed cream soups	from-scratch soup base with flour, butter, milk and added flavor (celery, chicken, etc.)	organic ingredients, homemade soup base and freeze
peanut butter	peanut butter without hydrogenated oils, added sugar	Natural nut butters (almond, cashew are good)
frozen chicken nuggets	from-scratch chicken nuggets	homemade nuggets with real chicken coated with panko or ground almonds
boxed cereal	cereal made with whole grain, no added sugar, no BHT	steel cut oats, homemade granola
commercial breadcrumbs	from-scratch organic bread, rolled oats, crushed bran cereal	almond flour

Chapter 4: The Kitchen Makeover

The pantry clean-out

Creating an organized pantry is the first step to stress-free meal preparation. The best way to tackle the pantry is to take everything out. Set all items on a kitchen island or table and then wipe down your shelves. You'll want to check your expiration dates first. Toss anything that is expired. I like to create zones in my pantry. Use one shelf for grains, pasta and rice; one shelf for breakfast items; one shelf for baking items (like flours and baking powder); and one shelf for canned food. Since I buy a lot of items in bulk, I like to store a lot of food, like rice and quinoa, in large, glass mason jars. Use a label maker to create a label for each jar.

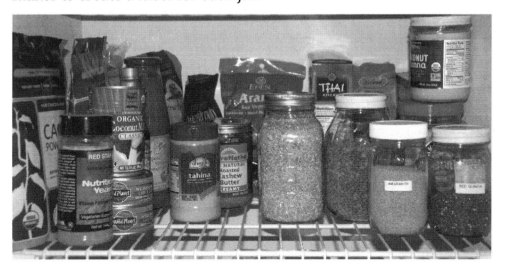

BEYOND THE BASICS

You may want to consider getting panty organizers like a canned food rack, shelf dividers or pull-out drawers once you've organized your space.

Next, start reading those labels. If a particular food item has one of the Nasty 9 ingredients, consider what you will do with that item. If it's a staple in your family's diet, consider finding a cleaner version. You can either toss the item now or finish it and decide not to purchase that brand anymore. If an item is something special and just used on occasion, you can either find cleaner versions or just not purchase it anymore. Most of the time, you will be able to find another healthier option of a particular food. It may be more expensive, but you are worth it and so is your health!

Some food items may be so full of chemicals that you'll have to accept the fact that you shouldn't buy that item anymore. This may upset some members of your family. This is where an open discussion about feeding our bodies with nourishing food will be handy. (See Chapter 9, Getting Family Members on Board for more tips.)

Healthier fats and oils

One of the staples in the "Standard American Diet" (SAD) pantry is **Vegetable Oil.** This is one of those items that **must go** in order to preserve your health. But why?

It's important to maintain a proper ratio of omega 3, 6 and 9 fatty acids in our bodies. The SAD leans very heavily on the Omega-6 and -9 fatty acids. Too many omega-6 fatty acids can cause inflammation, clogged arteries, heart disease and an increased risk of cancer. The average ratio of omega-6 to omega-3 fatty acids in Americans is between 10:1 and 25:1! This is definitely considered the danger zone. The ratio should be 4:1. This is mostly because of the high use of vegetable oils and the corn and soybean oils added to so many processed foods. For example, the ratio of corn oil is 83:1! Fats are made up of saturated, monounsaturated and polyunsaturated fats. The higher the content of saturated fats, the more stable that fat is and also resistant to breaking down or oxidizing when heated. Oils high in polyunsaturated fats will break down quickly when heated and cause oxidative stress to the body.

The most stable cooking fats

1. Ghee

Ghee is my favorite cooking oil. It is essentially clarified butter with the milk solids removed. It was traditionally used in India for Ayurvedic cooking. I use it the most because it has wonderful health benefits (only if you get grass-fed ghee) and has a rather high smoke point. Ghee is rich in the fat soluble vitamins A, D and K2. It is also rich in CLA (conjugated linoleic acid), the essential fatty acid found almost exclusively in grass-fed animals, which is now believed to protect against cancer, heart disease and type II diabetes.

Because the milk solids have been removed from ghee, this means that casein and lactose, the elements in dairy that many people are sensitive to, have been removed. Often, those with dairy sensitivities can tolerate ghee (consult a doctor before trying). The removal of the milk solids also allows you to use ghee at a higher temperature (up to 485 degrees). I use ghee for any cooking in a skillet like stir-fries, scrambled eggs, sautéed veggies, etc. You can find this in grocery stores and online, but it's also very easy to make on the stove or in the slow cooker.

2. Unrefined coconut oil

Not only does coconut have a wonderful flavor that goes great with any sweet baked good or even some savory dishes, especially Thai food, it also has wonderful health benefits. Sometimes cooking with this oil brings a coconut flavor to the dish, but I have found that the smell dissipates somewhat when cooking or is masked by other dominant flavors. Coconut oil has been said to aid in weight loss, support heart health, boost metabolism and benefit skin. It contains lauric acid, which has antibacterial, antioxidant and antiviral properties.

Unrefined virgin coconut oil is best used in low temperature cooking or baking. Refined coconut oil has a higher smoke point and almost no coconut flavor, but has less health benefits than raw coconut oil. Refined coconut oil is still a good option for occasional high-heat cooking like frying. When looking for coconut oil, make sure that it is not hydrogenated or treated with hexane.

3. Palm oil

Sustainably sourced palm oil is a great option for high-heat cooking and baking. It is made from the palm fruit, which is native to Africa. There has been a lot of controversy surrounding palm oil because many palm oil plantations have contributed to the decimation of the rainforest and the wildlife within it. However, you can source responsible and sustainably harvested palm oil, like Nutiva brand. I like to make my holiday cookies with palm oil, but it is high in Omega-6, so use sparingly.

4. Lard and bacon fat

Lard and bacon fat are also a healthier fat to cook with, but only if they are from pastured pigs. Lard is great to fry, sauté and bake with because of its high smoke point. Use in place of vegetable shortening for pie crusts and baked goods. Duck fat and tallow from beef are also excellent.

5. Grass-fed butter

Contrary to popular belief, high-quality grass-fed butter can be good for you. Although the mainstream media is slow to catch up, the link between saturated fats, cholesterol and poor heart health has been disproven. Our bodies need dietary cholesterol to function properly. So, long story short, don't worry about eggs or butter because your body (and brain especially) need cholesterol. Make sure you source good quality grass-fed butter. Organic, raw grass-fed butter is the best option. Organic Valley pastured butter is a great option too. Kerrygold butter is also a good choice and very affordable. Butter should be used in low temperature cooking since the smoke point is lower: 325 to 375 degrees.

Oils for low-heat cooking:

1. Extra virgin olive oil

Olive oil is a heart-healthy fat that contains beneficial antioxidants and has also been shown to have anti-inflammatory properties. It is best used for cold food (like salad dressing or drizzling over foods) but can be used in some low-heat cooking. Don't bring to a sizzle. Buy in a tin can or dark glass bottle.

Unfortunately, it has been discovered that some unsavory olive oil manufacturers have combined olive oil with cheap vegetable oils while still labeling the bottle as 100 percent olive oil, so make sure the olive oil you buy is pure, otherwise you may unwittingly be consuming unhealthy oils. Investigate the source!

2. Avocado oil

Avocado oil is another favorite oil of mine for cooking because it has such a high smoke point (475 to 520 degrees). However, it does contain a fair amount of polyunsaturated fats (PUFA) which, in excess, have been known to cause inflammation. Because of this, I don't use avocado oil as my everyday cooking oil, but it is a good choice for occasional use. You can also look for brands that offer avocado oil with low polyunsaturated fatty acid content like the Chosen Foods brand. I like to use this oil to make homemade mayonnaise.

Finishing or salad dressing oils:

1. Flax seed oil

High in omega-3s and Alpha Linolenic Acid (ALA), flax seed oil is a good oil for homemade salad dressings, but because of its high PUFAs, flax oil should not be used in cooking. Store in the fridge.

2. Macadamia nut oil

This oil is great for salad dressings and finishing a recipe. It has a low ratio of omega-6 fatty acids and some unique antioxidants. But do not cook or heat this oil or you risk it turning rancid. Store in the fridge. Can be pricey.

Unhealthy, man-made fats and refined seed oils:

1. Grapeseed oil

I know this one is going to be a big shocker for a lot of people, especially since grapeseed oil is constantly marketed as a healthy cooking oil. Well, the "health" of grapeseed oil (and most of the other oils on this list) is all based on misleading information and myths about cholesterol and heart health (I've explained this all above, so if you're skipping ahead, go back and read it if you really want to understand why grapeseed oil is not heart healthy!).

Grapeseed oil is about 70 percent omega-6 fatty acid (ratio of 676:1) which, as I explained above is way too much omega-6s. Too much omega-6 PUFAs causes inflammation, which is the true cause of heart disease. It can lead to other health problems like cancer and autoimmune disorders.

Oils that are high in polyunsaturated fats (PUFAs) like grapeseed oil are very fragile and therefore prone to oxidation. When oil oxidizes, it creates free radicals, which can also lead to cancer, inflammation, hormonal imbalance and thyroid damage. You can find cold-pressed grapeseed oil that may not be damaged during processing, but once you cook with it for a while, it will oxidize. I will use cold-pressed grapeseed oil for short cooking times, but not frequently.

2. Canola (rapeseed oil)

Canola is a marketing term and stands for Canadian oil or Canada oil, Low-acid. Unless organic and expeller-pressed, about 90 percent of canola oil is genetically modified. To create canola oil, one must take the crude oil that has been heat extracted from rape seeds (what canola oil is made from) and refine, bleach and deodorize it. Originally, rapeseed oil was used for industrial purposes. The fact that it is processed under high heat causes it to go rancid. A toxic solvent called Hexane is used to extract the oil from the rapeseeds. Cold-pressed and Organic Canola Oil does not go through the same damaging process and won't contain so many oxidized fats or trans fats.

3. Vegetable oil (soybean oil)

Although vegetable oil sounds healthy and natural because it seems like it's made of vegetables, about 99 percent of the time a bottle of vegetable oil is actually just soybean oil. You can even look at the ingredients in a bottle of vegetable oil next time you go to the grocery store . . . You'll see just one ingredient: soybean oil.

Soybean oil is 54 percent omega-6 (8:1 ratio), which like I discussed above is too much omega-6 and can lead to inflammation and health issues. Soybean oil is also likely to be GMO.

Soy is something that is best avoided or at least reduced in consumption unless it is fermented (like tempeh, natto or fermented soy sauce). I personally avoid soy for a few reasons. Soy is high in phytic acid and trypsin inhibitors, which means that it blocks the absorption of many vitamins, minerals and proteins. It also contains phytoestrogens that can mimic estrogen in the body and disrupt normal hormone function, which could possibly lead to increased cancer risk.

4. Corn oil

There is a popular misconception that corn is a vegetable. It is actually a grain. Corn originated and was bred from a tall grass-like plant that somewhat resembled wheat.

Corn oil has 58 percent omega-6 fatty acids, which is too high and can lead to inflammation. On top of that, corn is one of the most genetically modified crops in the US. About 88 percent (probably more) is GMO!

5. **Vegan butter substitutes and margarine**

These are a mix of canola and soybean oil. The Earth Balance brand is corn oil. Refer to statements above. Margarine is hydrogenated fat.

6. **Other industrial seed oils**

Other oils like Cottonseed, Sunflower, Safflower, Sesame and even Rice Bran Oil all contain high amounts of PUFAs and are very high in omega-6 fatty acids, not to mention the highly processed way they are created. Avoid altogether.

Note: High Oleic Safflower and Sunflower oils are okay in small amounts. They do contain the good monounsaturated fats. Choose high oleic over linoleic and refined oils.

Storing your oils

The causes of oxidative damage to cooking oils are heat, oxygen and light; therefore, keep them in a **cool, dry, dark place** and make sure to screw the lid on as soon as you're finished using them. Buy smaller bottles that you intend to use within a few months.

Safer sweeteners

Hopefully, by now you realize it's time to give up your little pink, blue or yellow packets of "sugar." Giving up sugar can be hard, but the energy you'll get from having balanced blood sugar will be so rewarding. I hardly ever use sugar now, so when I do taste something sweetened, I can only have a little because it tastes too sickly sweet. Your palate changes once you clean up your diet. Lowering the amount of sugar you consume can create vast improvements in your health. Think about all the places we found sugar hiding in Chapter 2. While these sweeteners may be healthier than artificial ones, they are still metabolized in the body by the liver and increase blood sugar levels, which can lead to insulin resistance, weight gain and diabetes. ALL sugar should be consumed as a condiment in the smallest serving possible.

Common table sugar is made up of glucose and fructose. Once in the body, the two split up and go their separate ways. Glucose is the body's main form of energy. It is immediately used or stored as fuel for later. But fructose can only be processed by the liver. There, it acts like fat. It's not used by the body for energy. Too much sugar can cause serious health problems and cavities. Some doctors advise that children have no more than four teaspoons of sugar per day and 6 for adults. So if you're starting your day with a typical bowl of cereal and skim milk, you're looking at an average of 22 grams or 5.5 teaspoons of sugar just at breakfast alone.

Maple syrup

Made from the sugary sap of maple trees, maple syrup contains a small amount of minerals, especially manganese and zinc. It's still two-thirds sucrose, so consume in very small amounts. Grade B syrup contains more antioxidants and is made from a late harvest. Make sure you buy real maple syrup and not maple-flavored syrup.

Raw honey

Honey contains antioxidants and trace amounts of vitamins and minerals.[35] It has slightly less harmful effects on metabolism than sugar.[36] Look for raw, unheated, pure honey from a local beekeeper. Once heated or pasteurized, it loses its healthful properties.

Coconut palm sugar

Coconut sugar is made by extracting the sugary liquid or sap and letting the water evaporate. It contains a small amount of fiber and nutrients and is low on the glycemic index. It's 35 to 45 percent fructose, which is still high. Consume with caution.

Sucanat

Sucanat stands for Sugar-Cane-Natural. It's simply dehydrated, freshly squeezed sugar cane juice. It has a rich molasses taste. This is a great substitute for brown sugar and can stand in for sugar in many recipes.

Molasses

Molasses is a delicious by-product that is extracted during the sugar cane refining process used to make sugar crystals. Sugar cane is crushed to remove the juice, which is then boiled vigorously. Machines utilize centrifugal force to extract the sugar crystals from the syrup. The remaining syrup becomes molasses. Contains trace amounts of vitamins and minerals.

Stevia

Stevia is extracted from the leaves of the plant. It is many hundred times sweeter than sugar. It has no calories and can lower blood pressure and blood sugar levels. Stevia can have a bitter aftertaste and you'll want to find a brand that hasn't been bleached or over-processed.[37,38]

Xylitol

Xylitol is a sugar alcohol with 2.4 calories per gram. It has some benefits for dental health, reducing the risk of cavities and dental decay.[39] Xylitol doesn't raise blood sugar or insulin levels either, but it can cause digestive distress if too much is consumed.[40]

Erythritol

Erythritol is found naturally in certain fruits, but the product you'll find in stores is made via an industrial process. It doesn't appear to raise blood sugar or insulin levels. Sugar alcohols can cause digestive issues when consumed in large amounts, so start with a small amount first. At .24 calories per gram, it's a very low-calorie sweetener. I don't deem this one to be as healthy because of the processing methods, but when consumed in small amounts, it doesn't have adverse health effects.[41]

Pure cane sugar

If you're looking for plain sugar, make sure the bag says "Pure Cane Sugar" on the label. Typically, store-brand sugar is genetically modified sugar beets. Use in extreme moderation.

Agave syrup

I'm not a fan of agave syrup for two reasons: it's 70 to 90 percent fructose and it's highly processed. It is low on the glycemic index, however, because of its high fructose content. Agave is much worse than regular table sugar.

HEALTH COACH TIP

The glycemic index (GI) is a measure of how quickly foods raise blood sugar levels. Glucose is given a GI of 100 and if a food has a GI of 50, then it raises blood sugar half as much as pure glucose.

Foods you can stop buying:

Normally I don't like to tell my clients not to eat something, but some things don't belong in our precious bodies. I shake my head when I read what's in some of these products and wonder how these manufacturers can sleep at night.

Soy products

Soy is a protein that is very hard to digest. Soy is high in phytic acid and trypsin inhibitors, which means that it blocks the absorption of many vitamins, minerals and proteins. It also contains phytoestrogens that can mimic estrogen in the body and disrupt normal hormone function, which could possibly lead to increased cancer risk. If it's not organic, it is probably GMO. Stick with fermented soy like tempeh, natto and soy sauce, and consume as a condiment.

Vegetable oils

Oils such as soybean, corn, cottonseed and canola are GMO oils that have an inflammatory effect on the body. Soybean oil is 54 percent omega-6, which is too high and can lead to inflammation and health issues like clogged arteries, heart disease and an increased risk of cancer. The average ratio of omega-6 to omega-3 fatty acids in Americans is between 10:1 to 25:1! That is well into the red zone.

Coffee creamers

Certain creamers on the market today lack any real food ingredients whatsoever. They consist of hydrogenated soybean or cottonseed oil (trans fats), gels, gums and carrageenan. Some flavors even contain artificial sugars, colors and preservatives. Avoid at ALL cost. Use real cream, milk or half-and-half or, for a non-dairy option, coconut milk or MCT Oil.

Bottled water

Most bottled water is tap water. It's contained in a plastic vessel that could very well be leaching Bisphenol A (BPA) or other synthetic estrogens like Bisphenol F or S. Plus, it's expensive and fills our landfills. (See Chapter 12 for more information on BPA and plastics.) Use a refillable stainless steel or glass bottle for your filtered water.

Juice and juice boxes

These seem healthy, as they are made from fruit. But juice can contain just as much sugar as soda. Juice doesn't contain the fiber necessary to slow the insulin spikes from consuming so much sugar at once. Whole fruit, an apple with its skin for example, is the better fiber- and vitamin-rich alternative. Juice boxes are convenient for kids, but they definitely don't need more sugar in their diet and a reusable bottle of water is much better for them. Some juices contain added sugar, artificial colors and preservatives, so check the label if you are purchasing juice and look for "no added sugar" or other additives.

Salad dressings

It's super easy to make a quick homemade dressing and sometimes you can get away with just a splash of Balsamic vinegar and extra virgin olive oil. Store-bought dressings are primarily made with soybean or canola oil, high-fructose corn syrup and lots of chemical preservatives and emulsifiers to keep the oil from separating. Check out the recipe section for some quick dressing ideas.

Artificial sweeteners

As discussed in the Nasty 9 section, those pink, blue and yellow packets should be avoided at all cost. These are all chemical-based sweeteners that destroy your health. Stick to real sugar.

Microwave popcorn

This product carries three major risks. First, there's the bag. The lining contains Perfluorooctanoic acid (PFOA), a dangerous chemical that persists in the environment. It's known to cause developmental issues, infertility and cancer in lab animals. Then, there are hydrogenated oils on the popcorn, along with TBHQ, propyl gallate and artificial flavors. Lastly, the popcorn kernels themselves could have been grown with pesticides and could even be contaminated by GMOs. Make your own in the microwave in a paper bag or on the stovetop. See the recipes section for some fun ideas!

Sports drinks

Most sports drinks on the market today are filled with stabilizers; citrates that can cause tooth erosion; dextrose (GMO corn); lots of sugar or artificial sugars like sucralose and acesulfame potassium; and artificial colors. A 12-ounce serving contains 21 grams of sugar or 5.25 teaspoons of sugar. Too much sugar can actually dehydrate you. A better alternative is plain water, pure coconut water, a banana or green juice with celery.

Frozen prepared meals, sandwiches and breads

Take a look at the list of ingredients contained in some of these "food" items. All of them contain partially hydrogenated oils, MSG, soybean oils, soy flours, sorbates (preservatives), HFCS and even artificial colors. This is a chemical concoction and not real food. There are healthier frozen meals from brands like Amy's and Helen's Kitchen, but it's best to just make yourself a quick breakfast or salad for lunch. See the recipe section.

Margarine, butter sprays and spreads

I can't believe these things are still on the market! They consist of partially hydrogenated oils, preservatives, emulsifiers and artificial colors. Not even close to real butter. You can buy sprays of coconut and avocado oil now.

Boxed cake mixes and canned frosting

Boxed cake mixes contain bleached flours, hydrogenated oils, aluminum phosphates, propylene glycol and artificial flavors and colors. Canned frosting is worse with more partially hydrogenated oils, corn syrup, caramel coloring and preservatives that can keep this product shelf-stable for years. A homemade cake is nothing more than flour, butter, sugar, eggs, baking soda and natural flavorings. Frosting is butter, sugar and maybe a splash of milk. Both are really easy to make.

Soft drinks

I know this is going to be hard, but I have faith—you can do this! Sodas are full of added sugar (in the form of either HFCS or artificial sugars that stimulate your appetite), phosphoric acid, caramel coloring, caffeine and preservatives. Diet soft drinks are particularly devastating to your health because of the dangers of the artificial sugars (see the Nasty 9). Phosphoric acid can erode tooth enamel and may also cause calcium loss in bones.[42] Caramel color IV (sulfite ammonium caramel, acid-proof caramel) contains both sulfites and ammonium compounds. There have been several human and animal studies conducted on caramel coloring. Some studies found that caramels produced with ammonium could inhibit the metabolism of B6, reduce white blood cell count or soften feces. In addition, animal studies showed possible carcinogenic effects. In 2011, the Center for Science in the Public Interest formally petitioned the U.S. FDA to revoke sections of legislation: " . . . which authorize the use in foods of caramel colorings that are produced by means of an ammonia or ammonia-sulfite process and contain 2-methylimidazole and 4-methylimidazole, both of which are carcinogenic in animal studies." Some soft drinks contain high doses of 4-methylimidazole, which are compounded by the numerous soft drinks some people consume in one day. Check out my following tips to wean yourself off soda.

How to ditch the soda habit

The consumption of soft drinks has increased **500 percent in the last 50 years**, according to the U.S. Department of Agriculture. Drinking soda increases your obesity risk by 60 percent, yet soda manufacturers reward you for drinking soda with cool gift cards and prizes. Schools are promoting this in the classroom to win popsicle parties![43]

I have many family members, friends and clients who are completely addicted to soda. Some just like the bubbles every now and then. Most of them are realizing the detrimental effects that drinking soda on a regular basis can have. Some experience pain in the abdomen, some get jittery, and others are obese. There are many studies linking soda to obesity.[44] Sugar-sweetened drinks increase the risk of obesity, diabetes, heart disease and gout. A 22-year study of 80,000 women found that those who consumed a can per day of a sugary drink had a 75 percent higher risk of gout than women who rarely had such drinks.[45] Researchers found a similarly elevated risk in men.[46] The phosphoric acid in colas and coffee also interfere with calcium absorption. This can cause brittle bones and deficiencies.

And then there's the caffeine. Colas have anywhere from 34 to 57 milligrams of caffeine in a 12-ounce serving, depending on the brand. Now, that's not as much caffeine as your typical latte from the corner coffee shop that contains around 75 milligrams per 12-ounce serving, but most people are drinking two to three colas per day. Caffeine has its own set of problems. Yes, it can boost metabolism and provide some laser-focused brain function, but there's a catch. Excess caffeine, anything over 150 to 200 milligrams per day, stimulates the central nervous system and kicks your body into fight-or-flight mode. This disrupts your stress hormones and can set you up for an increase in body fat. Your liver releases blood sugar in response to the perceived stress, your pancreas churns out insulin to balance out the blood sugar levels and this repeated action causes insulin resistance or pre-diabetes.

A typical 20 ounce soda contains 15 to 18 teaspoons of sugar and upward of 240 calories. A 64 ounce fountain cola drink could have up to 700 calories. Most soda is sweetened with GM aspartame or GM high-fructose corn syrup, both of which bring more health concerns to the table.

It can be hard to give up this habit, especially if you've been drinking soda for a long time. Most people like soda for the fizz. The carbonation provides the bubbles many yearn for.

Try these ideas to satisfy your soda cravings:
- Sparkling water can provide that fizz you seek; add in lemon, lime or orange slices or cranberry juice.
- Try Perrier or club soda with lime.
- Taper down slowly so you don't get a headache from caffeine withdrawal. Remove only one soda per day.

- Add in a cup of green tea or black tea for a smaller caffeine buzz.
- Switch from diet cola to regular. Then taper the amount of regular colas each day.
- Try Kombucha, a fermented tea that has a slight fizz and great health benefits.
- Purchase your own home carbonation system, like a SodaStream. However, make your own flavorings because their pre-packaged products are full of the same chemicals you need to avoid in soda.
- Try sweet or unsweetened tea.
- Purchase a reusable glass or stainless steel bottle and fill it up with tea or water at home.
- Really got to have that cola taste? Virgil's brand sodas are made naturally without caffeine or preservatives, but they contain a high amount of sugar, so limit your consumption.

The fridge makeover

Every once in a while you have to clean your fridge and what a better time than when you're cleaning up your diet. I'm sure you'll find a container of something that resembles a science experiment or a condiment from the last decade. So, first things first, remove all of the items. Start with the door and check the dates on your condiments. Toss everything that is expired and anything with mold growing around the edges. Even if a food item has a tiny bit of mold on the rim, root threads may have invaded the jar completely, so into the trash it goes!

Work your way from the top shelf down, removing each item, inspecting the label for the Nasty 9, smelling contents for "off" smells and tossing any non-nutritious items. Use this opportunity to clean the fridge. Remember to recycle those glass jars!

Clean the inside of the refrigerator every few months with 1 tablespoon of baking soda dissolved in a quart of water.

HEALTH COACH TIP

Keep a wipe-off board on your fridge and write down when you run out of something. Simply take a photo with your smart phone and head to the store. Voila! Your shopping list! Free phone apps, such as *Out of Milk*, can help, but it takes time to type in your lists.

How to store your food properly

Americans tend to throw out about 25 percent of the food in their fridges, either because of spoilage or because they don't have a plan for it. Uneaten food is the single largest component of municipal solid waste.

The key to avoiding spoilage is two-fold: have a food plan and store the food properly.

When you come home from the grocery store, prep your hardier vegetables for the current week's meals. If you need diced carrots for a soup or shredded cabbage for a slaw, go ahead and do this task as soon as you get home from the grocery store. Hardier root vegetables, green beans, onions and some tropical fruits can be cut up in advance and placed in damp cloths or glass storage containers, but don't wash berries or tender lettuces until you're ready to eat them.

Where in the fridge do I store the food?

Door

This is the warmest part of the fridge, where the temperature can be a degree or two warmer than the main compartment, so it's not a good home for anything highly perishable, like milk. Use the door's shelves for the collection of condiments you've amassed while perfecting your pad thai and the six jars of various types of mustards. Pasteurized juice can go here too. Butter can go in the covered compartment at the top.

Top shelf

This is the second-warmest area of the fridge. Put yogurt, nut-milks, leftovers and anything ready-to-eat up here. The back of the fridge tends to be coldest, so store your highly perishable items in the back.

Meat and cheese drawer

If you have one, this can be the designated home for your deli meats and cheese, where it's relatively warm. (Cheese, incidentally, can find many happy homes in the fridge, like the butter compartment.)

Middle shelf

This area tends to be a bit colder, so this is where eggs and milk should go, since this is where the temperature is most consistent in your fridge.

Bottom shelf

Keep raw meat and seafood here, in their original packaging, and toward the back, where it's coldest. If you buy a lot of meat and are concerned about drippy raw chicken juices contaminating fruits and vegetables in the drawers below (a valid concern), keep a separate plastic bin on this shelf devoted to uncooked meat. Bonus: Cleanup is easy if things do get messy.

Drawers and bins

Here's where things get a little complicated. Fruits and vegetables belong here, where refrigerator humidity levels are highest. But different produce requires different levels of moisture. Certain fruits emit ethylene, a gas that accelerates rotting in vegetables.

Your best bet is to keep fruits and vegetables separated. Keep fruit in the lowest-humidity drawer, often marked "Crisper," with the vent open, which allows more air to come in. Vegetables can tolerate more humidity, so keep the vent on this drawer closed, which keeps air from circulating and holds moisture in.

The freezer makeover

Follow the same steps included in the fridge makeover, but this time, take an inventory of everything. Note how many bags of frozen peas you have and how many pounds of ground beef are present. Toss anything that is covered in ice as it has been "freezer-burned" and won't taste good when cooked.

The freezer is a good place to store nuts and nut flours you don't use very often as well as ginger and soup bones for making stock.

Create a spreadsheet of the number of pounds of ground beef, pork chops, roasts, etc., the date you froze them, and what shelf they're located on. Put this list on your freezer door or tape it inside.

Helpful kitchen tools & gadgets

Being successful at whole food eating means having a stocked, clean kitchen and a plan. This requires certain systems to be in place. I'm going to show you how to create these systems.

It's important to keep your kitchen clean so you can walk in and prepare meals quickly. I like to use the "clean as you go" method. My mom can whip up a full meal with meat and three sides in twenty minutes, but the kitchen looks like a tornado whipped through once she's finished. I like to clean as I go when cooking, which can slow you down a bit, but items like a food processor are much easier to clean if you give them a quick rinse right after you use them. Find a method that works for you, but do clean up right after your meal. Kids as young as four years old can help carry plates to the sink. My children are old enough now to put the clean dishes away, and we put this duty on their chore charts to earn points for things like extra TV time or a movie night.

Having the right tools and appliances can make preparing healthy meals a tad easier as well. Here are some of my favorites:

Sharp knives. I say sharp because you can cut yourself very easily with a dull knife that can slide or slip off of food and onto your fingers. Use the honing tool that came with your knife set and sharpen your knives regularly.

Salad spinner. This is great for washing and drying all those greens veggies you'll be eating now.

High-powered blender. A few brands of high-powered blenders on the market can take on the task of blending smoothies, nuts and seeds. Good ones to check out include Ninja, Vitamix and Blendtec.

Large cutting boards. Wood cutting boards are best, but a couple of plastic ones are OK as well. Avoid cutting boards treated with Microban® or anti-bacterial agents, like triclosan.

Quality cookware. Options: cast iron, stainless steel, copper, ceramic.

Slow-cooker. This handy tool is a must for those busy nights.

Bamboo spoons, spatulas. Those plastic spoons could be leaching plasticizers and chemicals into your food. Stick with natural materials.

Food processor. Great for making granola bars, energy bites, cookies, nut butters, cauliflower rice and more.

Stand or hand mixer. Essential for whipping eggs, batters, homemade marshmallows (my favorite) and much more.

Beyond the Basics:

Instant pot. This electric pressure cooker is new to the home cooking scene but is quickly becoming a family favorite because it cuts cooking time in half, sometimes less. I can make creamy risotto in 6 minutes and roast a whole chicken in 15 minutes.

Spiralizer. This is a trendy new item that is used for making spiral vegetable pastas like zucchini pasta and cucumber noodle salad. Honestly, that's all I've used mine for, but if you need to stay away from flour pasta, this tool makes quick work of veggie pasta and it's fun too!

Having the right tools on hand can cut preparation and cooking time considerably. Grab a coupon and head to Kohl's or Bed, Bath & Beyond and treat yourself to a fun, new gadget.

Step Three:

The Tools

Chapter 5: Whole Food Transformations

I had the pleasure of working with three families to go through the steps outlined in this book as I was writing it. I taught them how to read ingredient labels and sent them healthy swap and shopping lists. It was an eye-opening experience for them as they went through the changes and swaps.

The Rightmyer Family

Becca and her family live in Lexington, Kentucky. She was a health coaching client of mine in 2013 and lost 35 pounds! She wanted to learn more about eating whole foods and help her husband who was diagnosed with high cholesterol. I taught her how to read ingredient labels, how to switch out her non-nutritious favorites and ditch her soda habit. She had this to say about the process:

"Having been coached by Cindy before, I thought there wasn't much that I needed to learn. I also was scared that the food would taste bad and be too difficult to prepare. I was wrong! The information that Cindy provided to our family has changed my entire way of looking at food. The switch to real food was both simple and tasty! All it requires is a bit more time to really read the ingredients on the foods you buy. I find myself doing it on EVERYTHING now. Just like any lifestyle change, it's a discipline. You have to continue to work at it and have checks and balances in place. You also have to extend grace to yourself because everyone has bad days."

Becca found brands that she could trust, and shopping trips are much easier now. She says that the healthier food actually tastes better, and she now knows which levers to pull when any weight starts to creep back on. Check out Becca's before and after photo!

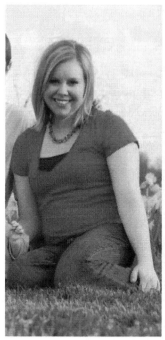
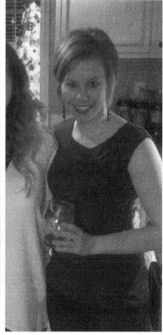

Before   After

The Crummett Family

The Crummetts live in Northern Virginia and have two young girls. The mom's main health concerns were allergies, asthma, frequent illnesses and low energy. She wanted to take on this change because she was at a pivotal point in her life and felt that it wasn't too late to establish healthy habits for her children. She started to read labels and went shopping for healthy swaps her entire family would approve of. She has experienced an increase in energy and more restful sleep. It's been a slow process for them, but they are making improvements and want to keep adding new healthy foods and habits into their lives. Check out some of their new snacks and sweetener.

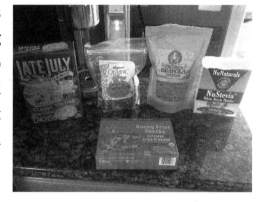

The Kline Family

The Klines live in Northern Virginia and have two teenage children. Several family members were suffering from skin conditions and eczema. Carolyn has been a label reader for quite a while, but that didn't always mean she bought healthy, unprocessed foods.

She shared this with me, "I have realized that when I eliminate processed foods I feel so much better. I have more energy and can focus more—my brain feels more awake. Also, removing processed sugar from my diet has eliminated my sugar cravings. This journey has made me realize that what I eat can hurt or help me, so I'm reading labels more often. My family is reading them too. I am making healthier purchases and preparing healthier meals as a result of being made aware of what processed foods were doing to me."

Carolyn's husband replaced his breakfast cereal with vegetable and fruit smoothies and no longer has mid-morning food cravings. Their daughter is more aware of what she puts in her body through the food choices she is making.

You can do this too with your family. Have a family meeting and talk openly about what changes you could make and how everyone can work together to support one another. Discuss what you should do first and what healthy habits you could add to your routines. Perhaps you could start having green smoothies in the morning or cook dinner together as a family. Starting a garden is another great way to get the whole family involved. Don't overcomplicate it. Start small with a simple tomato plant, lettuce and fresh herbs.

Chapter 6: Your First Real Food Shopping Trip

The first time I went shopping after learning about the Nasty 9 ingredients and what foods I needed to find healthier swaps for, it took me two hours! I spent a lot of time reading labels, putting boxes back on the shelf and just being plain disgusted at how so many foods were filled with chemical preservatives and colors. But once I found brands that I could trust and healthier versions of our family favorites, shopping trips became much quicker. Sometimes I don't even venture into two-thirds of the grocery store because I find what I need in fresh produce and the organic section and get out!

The Environmental Working Group (ewg.org) releases an annual updated report that identifies foods in the conventional, non-organic food supply that contain the highest number of pesticide residues. The worst offenders, which were nicknamed the **"The Dirty Dozen,"** include:

The Dirty Dozen Plus	*The Clean 15*
Apples	Avocado
Peaches	Sweet corn (non-GMO)
Strawberries	Pineapples
Nectarines	Cabbage
Grapes	Sweet peas (frozen)
Celery	Onions
Spinach	Asparagus
Sweet bell peppers	Mangoes
Cucumbers	Kiwi
Cherry tomatoes	Papaya
Snap peas	Eggplant
Potatoes	Grapefruit
+ Hot peppers	Cantaloupe
+ Kale, Collard greens	Cauliflower
	Sweet potatoes

Conventionally grown items on the **"Clean 15"** list are generally lower in pesticides. "More than 90 percent of cabbage, asparagus, sweet peas, eggplant and sweet potato samples had one or fewer pesticides detected," the EWG report says. "Of the 'Clean 15' vegetables, no single sample had more than five different chemicals, and no single fruit sample from the 'Clean 15' had more than five types of pesticides detected."

Exposure to pesticides is linked to numerous health concerns. They contain chemicals classified as obesogens, which are endocrine disrupting chemicals that cause our bodies to store fat and increase the number of fat cells. Others expand the size of fat cells and still others influence appetite, cravings, fullness and how well the body burns calories.

REAL FOOD Shopping List

Condiments and oils

- Honey (raw unfiltered)
- Maple syrup (dark grade B has more nutrients)
- Dijon mustard
- Organic ketchup
- Organic BBQ sauce
- Organic tomato sauce
- Organic salsa
- Almond, cashew butter
- Pasture-raised butter, ghee
- Organic peanut butter (use sparingly)
- Raw apple cider vinegar (Bragg's)
- Balsamic vinegar
- Red wine vinegar

- Coconut liquid aminos
- Coconut oil (Unrefined Extra Virgin)
- Olive oil (cold-pressed organic extra virgin)

Nuts, Seeds & Dried Fruit:

- Almonds
- Brazil nuts
- Cashews
- Walnuts
- Flaxseed
- Pumpkin seeds
- Sunflower seeds
- Cranberries
- Raisins
- Dates

I rate **almonds** as the healthiest of the nuts listed because they are a great source of Vitamin E.

I rate **pumpkin seeds** as the healthiest of all listed seeds. They're rich in protein and carbohydrates and lower in fat compared to the others. They also contain several essential nutrients, including vitamin K and zinc. Zinc is an important nutrient and is only present in some healthy, whole foods.

HEALTH COACH TIP

Purchase raw, unsalted nuts if you can find them. That way you can control the amount of salt you're consuming, if any.

Fruits

(D) On the Dirty Dozen. Buy the organic version if possible

- Apples (D)
- Apricots (occasional)
- Bananas (occasional; high glycemic index)
- Blueberries
- Cranberries
- Grapes (D)
- Lemon and limes for cooking
- Plums
- Peaches (D)
- Pineapple
- Raspberries
- Strawberries (D)
- Watermelon

I rate organic **strawberries** as the healthiest of all listed fruits in terms of nutrient content. They contain vitamin C, manganese, fiber, iodine, potassium, folate, vitamins B2, B5 and B6, omega-3 fatty acids, vitamin K, magnesium and copper.

They also contain phenolic compounds, which are powerful anti-oxidants. They are heart-healthy, anti-cancer and anti-inflammatory fruits. Be careful to buy organic fruits to avoid residual pesticides. Pesticides can't be washed off, unfortunately!

Remember the glycemic index when it comes to fruit. Low-GI foods cause a slow and gradual rise in blood glucose; high-GI foods break down quickly, causing a sudden spike in blood glucose. A diet based on low-GI foods can be beneficial to health, particularly for those struggling with weight control or diabetes management.

Vegetables

(D) Dirty Dozen, buy the organic version if possible

- Asparagus
- Avocado
- Beets
- Broccoli
- Cabbage (purple or green)
- Carrots
- Cauliflower
- Celery (D)
- Collard greens (D)
- Green beans/peas
- Garlic
- Kale (D)
- Onions
- Red, yellow and orange peppers (D)
- Spinach (D)
- Salad mix of baby spinach and spring salad mix/field greens (D)
- Squash yellow
- Sweet potatoes
- Tomatoes
- Zucchini

I rate **dark green leafy vegetables** (including leafy herbs) as the healthiest of all listed vegetables. The nutritional value of these vegetables include high levels of fiber and high levels of a range of nutrients including beta carotene (precursor to Vitamin A), folate, iron and Vitamin K.

I try to buy most of my fruits and vegetables organic or locally grown. The closer they are grown to your home, the less anti-fungal agents are used on the product resulting in less toxins consumed. Visit LocalHarvest.org for a farmer's market near you.

HEALTH COACH TIP

Don't waste your money on those expensive vegetable washes at the store. You can rinse vegetables with water or add vinegar to a bowl with water and wash dirtier greens that way.

Meats/Protein

- Chicken (organic, free range)
- Eggs (organic, free range)
- Halibut
- Red meat—eat occasionally; lean, organic grass-fed (Venison)
- Salmon (wild caught, not farm raised)
- Sardines
- Scallops
- Flounder
- Turkey

I rate **sardines** as the best seafood. They are a small fish species occurring lower in the food chain and contain less bio-accumulated mercury. They are also rich in important nutrients like vitamin B12, selenium, vitamin D, phosphorous and calcium.

Don't be scared to try them. Just grill or pan-fry them with a squeeze of lemon juice. Generally, seafood is rich in concentrated omega-3 fatty acids and minerals such as iodine, zinc, magnesium and selenium.

Today's seafood presents a risk of mercury contamination and pathogenic bacteria. Smaller species of fish that are lower on the food chain (e.g. their food source is mainly plant-based) may contain lower levels of mercury, and are therefore considered to be safer choices. Wild caught is best.

Legumes

- Black beans
- Chickpeas
- Dried peas
- Kidney beans
- Lentils
- Lima beans
- Miso (organic)
- Pinto beans
- Soybeans (organic)
- Tempeh (organic)

I rate the healthiest legumes on this list as **kidney beans**, because they contain the most vitamins and minerals; notably folate, iron, fiber, phosphorous, copper and magnesium. Miso must rate a mention for its zinc content, because zinc is typically low in many Western diets.

HEALTH COACH TIP

Choose dried beans when you can or seek out BPA-free canned foods. Always rinse your canned beans to remove added sodium and wash away as much BPA as you can.

Whole Grains

(GF) Gluten-free grains

- Ezekiel whole grain bread
- Brown Rice Bread (GF)
- Barley
- Millet (GF)
- Oats (GF available)
- Quinoa (GF)
- Wild rice (GF)
- Rye
- Spelt
- Spinach pasta (whole wheat or GF Brown Rice)
- Whole Wheat pasta
- Buckwheat (GF)

I rate **oats** as the healthiest grain because they are rich in minerals, fiber and protein. Since oats may contain gluten, many people that can't have gluten foods are choosing Quinoa (pronounced keen-wah), which is a complete protein. Whole grains are healthy whole foods. Their outer husks contain healthy fats and the minerals we need (like chromium and selenium) to help digest the carbohydrate in the grain.

Dairy/Non Dairy

- Almond milk, unsweetened without carrageenan (make your own with raw soaked almonds and filtered water)
- Coconut milk (full-fat canned or unsweetened)
- Goat milk
- Raw cow milk (from a reputable farm)

Beverages

- Filtered spring water
- Organic vegetable juice
- Organic fruit juice specifically blueberry, cranberry and pomegranate juices. Buy in glass bottles and water down
- Coconut water
- Kombucha
- Apple cider vinegar diluted in water

Spices & Herbs

Have fun with spices and herbs and try new ones.

- Basil
- Cayenne pepper
  - high in vitamin A
  - helps fight and soothe inflammation
  - offers natural pain relief
  - promotes heart health
  - purifies the blood
  - increases sweating and fluid elimination
- Chili powder
- Cilantro
  - detoxifying
- Cinnamon
  - supports sugar and fat metabolism
  - regulates blood sugar and insulin in the body
  - has an impact on foods that regulate blood sugar and keeps your system steady
- Cumin
  - good source of iron and manganese
  - benefits digestive system

- Garlic
    - cleanses harmful bacteria, intestinal parasites and viruses from the body—especially from the blood and intestines
    - cleanses buildup from the arteries and lowers blood pressure in addition to having anti-cancer and antioxidant properties that help detoxify the body of harmful substances
- Ginger
    - healing spice
    - high in antioxidants
    - soothing to the stomach
    - stimulates circulation and sweating
- Himalayan sea salt
- Mustard seeds
    - rich in phyto-nutrients, minerals, vitamins and anti-oxidants
- Oregano
- Parsley
    - excellent source of Vitamin C, iodine, iron and other minerals
    - a diuretic that flushes the kidneys.
    - Avoid if breastfeeding, lowers your milk supply
- Pepper
- Peppermint
- Rosemary
- Thyme
- Turmeric
    - yellow powder used in Chinese medicine
    - anti-inflammatory

- improves liver function
- lowers cholesterol
- Vanilla

Herbs are some of the healthiest whole foods available. I rate the healthiest herbs on this list as **basil** and **mustard seeds,** both of which contain the greatest variety of vitamins and minerals. Adding fresh herbs to a meal is an easy way to boost the nutrient content.

Chapter 7: Saving Time and Money with Real Food

One of the first and biggest complaints I get from clients and friends is that buying "real" food is expensive. I will agree with that, but only to a certain extent. Grass-fed, pastured meats are more expensive than conventionally raised meats and some organic produce may be a bit higher than regular produce, but there are a lot of processed foods that are just as expensive as organic food and completely unnecessary.

My friend and farmer, Jesse Straight of Whiffletree Farm, says that people's true priorities are shown in how they spend their money and time. Jesse suggests that they have been habitualized into purchasing inexpensive industrial food. He recommends you review your entire family's budget when considering making changes to your food spending. You may have to keep an older car, refrain from annual vacations or dine out less when shopping for healthy, local, sustainable and ethical food. Jesse also suggests doing some of the work yourself. For example, he can cut up the chicken for you and charge you for that, or you can learn how to do it yourself and save a lot of money per pound. Learning how to render your own lard to replace expensive butter and olive oil can save you money too. Jesse recommends purchasing a used upright chest freezer and buying a pig or cow in bulk to save hundreds of dollars.

Meal Planning

If your evenings are currently crammed with afterschool activities and sports, then you'll need a plan. You can't wait to the last minute to prepare a meal, or you'll be forced to hit up the drive-through again.

I know we are all busy, but we have to shift our focus from fast and cheap to quick yet nourishing.

Planning can't begin until you know what everyone likes. Survey your family members and ask them what their favorite meals are. Then sit down with your spouse, think of your own favorite meals and start your planning.

Essentially meal construction in itself can be very simple. Simply **fry, bake, stew or poach a piece of good quality meat, fish or chicken. Then steam, roast or boil a side of fresh or frozen vegetables**, making sure to add a good amount of healthy fat in the form of butter, ghee, lard, coconut oil or olive oil in the process for taste, energy and health.

Sometimes planning a whole week's menu can be a daunting task, and honestly, I get a hankering for something different than what I had originally planned. So, I usually will plan 2 to 3 days or even just 24 hours in advance. But whatever you do, always have a plan. You can write it down and stick it on the fridge or use a free app like *Food Planner* on your smart phone. I like to write mine on my mini whiteboard on the fridge. That way it's front of mind and easy for everyone to see.

There's always going to be one or two crazy nights where the kids have after-school activities or you have to work late. So, I always have a slow-cooker meal or quick soup planned for at least one meal per week. Breakfast for dinner is always a good bet, too, and it's ready in ten minutes. Don't forget to thaw your meats 24 hours in advance! It doesn't help to have a freezer full of meals if you forget to thaw them! Make sure you plan out your side dishes as well. I like to shop the farmer's market every weekend to get my fresh veggies for the week. You can also incorporate leftovers into another night's meal. For example, you could brown a big batch of ground beef or ground pork to use for dinner on two different nights. I keep a running log or "star" the meals my family likes and scratch out the ones that didn't make muster. We try a lot of new recipes in this family and sometimes they just don't turn out right. I have to keep a lot of backups on hand, like canned tuna or salmon. Or I whip up some eggs and we have breakfast for dinner when that happens!

Get the whole family involved and create a Meatless Monday, Taco Tuesday, Slow-Cooker Wednesday, 10-Minute Dinner Thursday and Fish on Friday meal plan.

Time-saving dinner tips:

- Choose a pasta, add a sauce and add 2 to 3 diced veggies.
- Slow cooker soup formula: Choose a bean, add two to four veggies, add a whole grain (brown rice, quinoa, barley, etc.) and fill with stock. Season with your favorite spices and add a protein if you want.
- Check out a YouTube video and learn how to cut up a whole chicken, which is cheaper than already cut up parts, and freeze. One whole chicken can carry you through three meals for a family of four:
    - one meal of legs and thighs
    - one meal with breast meat
    - a pot of chicken soup made from the back and bones and any leftover meat
- Roast your whole chicken in the oven, save your leftovers and make chicken salad for lunch or chicken tacos for another dinner that week. Always save your bones to make homemade stock (see recipe section). If you don't have time that night, freeze your bones.
- When you have the time, meal prep or cook a couple of meals on

the weekend. This cuts your time for meal prep during the week. Just add a side veggie and you have a complete meal!

- I plan the week's meals, then make anything ahead that I can on Sunday to make the week easier. This includes chopping veggies, roasting veggies, cooking rice, quinoa, etc.
- Cook once, eat multiple times. Examples:
  - roast two chickens on Sunday, so you'll have already cooked chicken to toss into quick meals all week long
  - cook a roast beef or pork tenderloin that's larger than you need so you can make the leftovers into fast dinners later on.
- Prep your slow cooker meals the night before if your mornings are too rushed.
- You can also precook 4 cups of rice, portion out 1 cup servings and place those in freezer bags. Pull out what you need and thaw overnight.
- Build freezer meals. Take a bag of frozen shrimp, frozen vegetables and frozen cooked rice and toss into a large skillet with a lid. Dinner will be ready in 20 minutes.

All of these tips can work together to make meal times easier, but you need to create a system to put them into place.

Here is my family's Menu Planning System. I created a list of our favorite meals and we rotate them, so we don't get bored.

Family Dinner Planning Menu	
Chicken	**Pork**
Chicken with sundried tomatoes and leeks	Pork tenderloin*
Chicken fajitas	Honey cashew pork *

Chicken tacos with peppers and onions*	Carnitas, tacos or BBQ pulled pork
Chicken jambalaya*	Pork chops
Chicken with lemon butter, capers*	
Chicken parmesan	**Fish**
Chicken nuggets*	White fish Veracruz*
Roast chicken	Baked salmon with pineapple salsa
Enchiladas*	Grilled salmon*
Pad thai*	Sautéed sea scallops
Grilled chicken salad	Fried flounder
BBQ chicken pizza*	Shrimp pad thai*
	Salmon croquettes*
Beef	Fish (cod) tacos with honey and cilantro
Meatloaf*	
Homemade Hamburger Helper*	
Meatballs with quinoa pasta*	**Soup**
	Beans and greens
Vegetarian	Beef chili
Salads	White chicken chili*
Portobello mushroom pizza*	Vegetable
Kale salad	Chicken noodle
Power salad*	Potato leek
Stuffed peppers	Butternut squash*
Quinoa stew*	Chicken enchilada soup (slow cooker)*
	Beef stew
Sides	Shrimp and corn chowder
Braised kale*	Chicken tortilla
Braised collards*	Gazpacho*
Braised bacon cabbage	
Spaghetti squash*	**Desserts**
Quinoa pilaf	Molten lava chocolate cake*
Quinoa tabbouleh*	Dates
Risotto	Fresh fruit
Steamed & pan-fried broccoli	

Flavor Profiles for Marinades, Sauces
Asian: ginger, Thai chiles, soy, tamari, garlic
Italian: EVOO, basil, oregano, thyme, rosemary, marjoram
Greek: garlic, lemon, EVOO, mint, parsley, dill
Mexican: cumin, onion, oregano, tamarind, jalapeno, cilantro, lime
Indian: turmeric, curry, coriander, garam masala, mustard seeds
Caribbean: lime, jerk seasoning, allspice, orange, pineapple, coconut
*Recipe can be found in the recipe section.

Stretching a meal to save you money

Chicken four ways

I buy whole chickens to cut up and use the way I want. I will usually roast a whole chicken every week. The first night we enjoy a breast, thigh or leg. Then I take all the meat off the bones and save it for future meals. I can use chopped chicken for chicken salad, larger pieces for chicken tacos, or thinly shredded meat for chicken noodle soup. I save the bones for making stock. If I don't have time to make stock that night, I put the bones in the freezer for when I do have the time.

Utilizing leftovers

In the recipe section, I have a recipe for pork tenderloin. I will usually make two tenderloins and the extra one will turn into my pork tenderloin cashew stir-fry another night that week. This method of cook once, eat twice makes it a breeze to get through a week's meals.

Thanksgiving is another great time to utilize leftover turkey meat. I will actually buy a turkey larger than what I need for the holiday. After the big meal, I debone the turkey. I put a combo of white and dark meat in quart and gallon-sized bags and freeze them. These can be made into soups, casseroles, enchiladas and tacos. I always save the carcass to make stock. Leftover stock can be frozen as well.

Money-saving tips in the kitchen

- Buy blocks of cheese instead of shredded cheese that has added stabilizers and cellulose. Use the food processor's shredding blade and then store in a glass container in the fridge.
- Stockpile when items go on sale (rather than menu planning and then shopping). Don't forget to check online sites like Amazon, Vitacost and Nutiva for sales on your favorite items.
- Ordering groceries online cuts down on impulse buys.
- Buy pantry items in bulk that have a long shelf life. Examples include: pasta, spaghetti sauce, canned fish, canned beans, chicken stock and grains. Meal plan around what's on sale and what you have coupons for while incorporating bulk items.
- Make more than you need for easy lunches and quick dinners in the future.
- Make sure to use all of what you buy, as wasting food is the biggest budget buster.
- Eat seasonally when it comes to produce, as prices on what's in season are usually better.
- Shop your local farmer's market. They often have fruits and vegetables cheaper than grocery stores, and you're supporting a local farmer!
- Always compare the price per unit when buying like items. Sometimes a bulk item may be more expensive than a packaged item.

Food preservation

What do you do when you have purchased too much produce or don't want to eat salad tonight? It's going to spoil soon! Here are some tips on preserving your food:

- Store nuts and nut flours in the fridge or freezer to keep their oils fresh and from going rancid.
- Fruit going bad? Wash berries and place on a cookie sheet and pop into the freezer until frozen. Then store in a freezer bag. For other fruit, wash and cut and do the same. Frozen bananas make great smoothies when frozen.
- Puree your fruit and save for making popsicles or homemade fruit roll-ups.
- For herbs like cilantro and parsley, freeze extras in a little bit of olive oil in ice cube trays. You can also place sprigs of rosemary or tarragon into a bottle of olive oil and make an infused oil for salad dressings.
- Some veggies like broccoli and cauliflower can be cut and frozen like the berries on a sheet pan. But some veggies don't stand up well to this method and it's best to cook them and then freeze. Try this with tomatoes, eggplant and zucchini.
- Some greens like spinach, kale and collards do best with being cooked first, like in a soup, and then frozen.
- For meat that is near its prime, wrap tightly with wax paper or parchment and seal in a plastic bag. This method is for meat that has not been frozen before. Make sure to get all the air out so you won't have freezer burn.
- For previously frozen meat, cook it first into a meatloaf, meatballs, chili or soup, and then freeze it.

Healthy eating budget-friendly tips

- Shop the farmer's market April through November when produce is in season; find one near you at LocalHarvest.org.
- Eat seasonally, choosing foods that are grown in season like apples in the fall, berries in early summer and greens in the spring. Buy those items in larger quantities when they're in season and freeze or can the extras.
- If you can't choose organic whole grains, go for whole wheat flour, brown rice, bags of beans in bulk, quinoa, barley and couscous (Costco is great for this).
- If you can't afford grass-fed beef, choose pork or poultry, because, by law, it can't have growth hormones added to it. Don't pay extra for pork or poultry with "hormone-free" on the label; it's federally prohibited to add hormones.
- Grow your own herbs and lettuce on your windowsill. It's easy even for apartment dwellers.
- Shop the bulk bins. Oats, nuts, grains, rice are usually cheaper in bulk.
- Always compare the price per ounce or pound (referred to as the Unit Price).
- Share one-third or half a cow or pig with a friend or neighbor. You can get a pastured animal for as low as 3 dollars per pound.
- Visit the websites of organic products like Horizon milk or Stonyfield yogurt and "Like" their Facebook pages. Almost all of them have $1 off coupons on their sites.
- Sign up for newsletters from your favorite healthy food purveyors:
- Vitacost has frequent sales and BOGO offers.
- Nutiva has a special every Tuesday and they also offer to send out emails.
- Costco has great deals on organic foods, like large bags of quinoa,

coconut oil, maple syrup and organic milk.

- Amazon offers "Subscribe & Save" deals.
- Whole Foods has sales every Friday.
- The biggest cost saver is planning. When you plan meals, you have a set goal for each night and you have a set plan for each veggie and protein you buy. Don't go to the store without a plan. Make a list of your favorite meals: chicken, pork, turkey, fish, beef, veggie and soup. Come up with at least twenty-five meals to keep in rotation with extras for variation.
- How often do you throw away bad produce from the bottom of your veggie bin? When you plan, you don't waste food, which saves you money.
- Cook once, eat two or three times. Make a double batch of tacos, chili, butternut squash soup, meatloaf—these freeze really well.
- Join a CSA or Community Supported Agriculture. $500 might seem like a lot to pay up front, but it will feed your family of four all summer through early November, and comes to about twenty dollars per week for local, organic food.
- Drink water instead of expensive juices and sodas that are detrimental to your health. Flavor water with fruit, orange slices or mint for a refreshing change of taste.
- Pack snacks like nuts, seeds, fresh fruit, beef sticks, nut butters and water in a reusable glass or stainless bottle when you're on the go so you won't be tempted to stop at a fast food joint or Starbucks.
- Eating out is expensive: fifty to sixty dollars for a family of four. That same amount could buy a pork shoulder, a couple of chickens, three pounds of ground beef and enough veggies for almost two weeks of food!
- You actually eat less when you feed your body nutrient-dense foods.

- Pack yourself a lunch for work. Utilize leftovers: power salad, soup in a thermos, homemade trail mix or granola bars for snacks.
- Save your scraps for making stock; just toss in a freezer bag. Or use your scraps to make compost for the garden.
- Consider skipping convenience items like shredded cheese. These products are cheaper in a block and don't have all the added anti-caking ingredients like cellulose or wood pulp.
- Consider washing your produce when you bring it home from the grocery store. Set up a prep area, wash vegetables (not berries) and do your pre-chop prep for the week's meals. This saves an incredible amount of time when it comes to preparing your dinners each night.
- Keep certain fruits away from certain veggies. For example: apples give off ethylene gas, which ripens bananas and avocados more quickly.
- Store citrus in the fridge to make it last longer.
- Store raw nuts, seeds and flours in the fridge to keep them from going rancid (especially almond flour).
- Eat less meat. Vegetables are inexpensive, and a cup of wild or brown rice with some stir-fried veggies is a super cheap dinner. Oatmeal for breakfast, a power salad for lunch and a couple of vegetarian nights per week can really cut costs.
- Grocery store organic brands are a good option and usually cheaper.

If you can't afford organic meats, your best options are to go for the hormone- and antibiotic-free options as a supplement to vegetarian protein sources like local eggs, beans and organic dairy products.

Chapter 8: Healthy Eating on the Road and Dining Out

In order to continue with your healthy, clean eating while away from home, it's good to do a bit of research and find where some healthier restaurants or grocery stores are so you can stay on track with your healthy habits. I always allow a few extra minutes to re-search my destination before we travel.

Eating healthy on the road

Got a road trip this year? Here are some tips on how to eat healthy on the road:

- Plug in your route on EatWellGuide.org, and it will give you a list of healthy food options along your route. Plug in your destination to get tons of local, organic food options where you'll be staying as well.
- Pack a cooler. Our kids get bored easily in the car and having go-to snacks on hand as well as lunches already packed means less stops, happy kids and getting to our destination quicker! Try these options:
  - bananas
  - apples
  - grapes
  - pre-made trail mix (nuts, seeds, dried fruit)
  - homemade granola bars
  - hummus with cut up cucumber
  - carrots and bell peppers
  - sandwiches for the kids
  - power salad
  - protein power balls

- o homemade granola
- o Newman's Own High Protein Pretzels
- o Nick's Beef Sticks
- o organic tortilla chips
- Bring refillable, reusable water bottles. Ditch the plastic bottles that fill up landfills and expose you to more BPA. Buy a glass or stainless steel bottle and refill it!

Eating healthy on a plane

Knowing a few secrets can get you by those pesky new TSA rules!
- Pack your breakfast in a baggie! I pack quick-cooking rolled oats, cinnamon, chia seeds, nuts and my homemade granola in a baggie. Once through security, I look for a coffee shop and get a cup of hot water and a spoon (almost always free). You can also add dried fruit like raisins, cranberries or apples to sweeten it up.
- Take a banana with a packet of almond butter.
- Bring a power salad. For every plane trip I took last year, I made a power salad in a small BPA-free plastic container. It had greens, a protein like quinoa, chickpeas or tuna fish, topped with sunflower seeds, diced avocado, chia seeds, chopped veggies like cucumber, bell peppers, and carrots, and a tiny container of homemade dressing. I stop by a café and grab a fork before getting on the plane.
- Pack dried fruit, dark chocolate-covered nuts, trail mix, granola, blueberries, raw pumpkin seeds, sunflower seeds, raw nuts and homemade granola bars for the kiddies.
- Don't forget water! Bring an empty refillable water bottle (stainless steel is best) and fill it up at a café soda fountain after you pass through security. It's important to have lots of water for dehydrating plane trips!

- Pack herbal teas. I love packing a baggie of my favorite herbal teas. You can usually get hot water on a longer plane trip. Some of my favorites include:
  - Peppermint for a pick-me-up or tummy troubles
  - Ginger is great for tummies as well
  - Vanilla rooibos
  - Honey lavender
  - Lemon
  - I always take Yogi Detox tea everywhere I go, which is made with dandelion root that helps to detoxify excess water and toxins from the body.

Eating healthy in a hotel

Book hotel rooms that have a mini-fridge. I like packing a few staples in my suitcase and then tossing a few local finds in the fridge.

- Stop by a local market and buy some string cheese, plain yogurt, nut butter, raw veggies, hummus and crackers.
- Bring baggies of quick-cooking oatmeal and make some hot water by running water through the hotel room coffee maker.
- Pack your protein powder or green powder and add water to a BlenderBottle for a quick breakfast shake. I make pre-made baggies of True Whey or Plant Fusion powder, powdered spiriulina, maca powder, raw cacao and chia seeds.
- Store fresh fruit like apples, oranges, grapes, berries and bananas in the fridge.
- Make sure you save some snacks for the car or plane ride home.

Eating healthy in a vacation home/condo (with a kitchen)

When taking a longer vacation in a home or condo, I like to call ahead to see what they have. That way I typically only need to pack a few extra essentials. Sometimes I'll pack a blender, some spices and a few of my favorite knives if traveling by car. I have even known a few of my healthier friends to pack blenders in their suitcase!

I plan out our route on EatWellGuide.org and find local restaurants, farmer's markets and even organic grocery stores to shop. I pack a cooler of some of our frozen pastured pork and grass-fed beef and plan out our meals for the week, which also includes some evenings out at a few local restaurants that cater to those looking for healthier foods.

Dining Out

Most restaurants today use pre-packaged, pre-marinated meats that are trucked in from food distributors. Most of them actually purchase their products from the same company like Sysco and US Foods. These foods can contain HFCS, trans fats, chemical preservatives and more ingredients listed in the Nasty 9. A restaurants' job is to create a meal that has enough fat, salt and sugar to keep you coming back for more. They will source inexpensive sweeteners, inflammatory GMO cooking oils and conventional meats in order to turn a profit. But knowing a few tricks can help you avoid some of these ingredients.

Most of the larger chain restaurants will put their menu online with the major ingredients listed. All fast food restaurants have to do this. That's how we know what the ingredients are in McDonald's and Chick-fil-A's French fries.

McDonald's French fries:

> Ingredients: Potatoes, Vegetable Oil (Canola Oil, Soybean Oil, Hydrogenated Soybean Oil, Natural Beef Flavor [Wheat and Milk Derivatives], Citric Acid [Preservative]), Dextrose, Sodium Acid Pyrophosphate (Maintain Color), Salt. Prepared in Vegetable Oil: Canola Oil, Corn Oil, Soybean Oil, Hydrogenated Soybean Oil with TBHQ and Citric Acid added to preserve freshness. Dimethylpolysiloxane added as an antifoaming agent.

Chick-fil-A French fries:

Potatoes (vegetable oil [canola oil, palm oil], disodium dihydrogen pyrophosphate [to promote color retention], dextrose), fully refined high oleic canola oil (TBHQ and citric acid added to preserve freshness and Dimethylopolysiloxane added as an anti-foaming agent).

The only real food in both of these is potatoes!

Guide to restaurant dining

- Make note of the healthy food items. Clear broth-based soups; raw or steamed vegetables; a plain, baked potato; and meats that are grilled, roasted or baked are usually healthier choices. Meals that are fried, breaded, creamy or crispy are generally high in calories, unhealthy fats or sodium.
- Check the restaurant's website before going there. Look for a page on their website that displays the nutritional information for their menu items. Make selections that are low in calories and fat but high in vitamins, minerals and other nutrients when possible.
- Plan your food consumption for the day accordingly. By limiting your calorie or fat consumption during the day, you may have more food options from which to choose without going over your fat and sodium allotment for the day.
- Note how many servings are in each portion of the menu item you select. If it contains multiple portions, share the meal with a friend or ask the server to box up half of the meal for you to take home.
- Avoid mindless nibbling before the meal. Many restaurants serve a basket of bread or a bowl of chips before the meal. Even though taking a few bites is harmless, be conscious about what

you eat so you do not eat more than you want to without realizing it. You can always refuse the bread basket!

- Ask the server for modifications. Many restaurants offer customers choices in the way the food is prepared or they will serve sauces on the side, so don't be afraid to ask for healthier alternatives.
- Stop eating when you feel full. Ask for your plate to be taken away or your food to be placed in a carryout container when you are finished, even if your dining companions are still eating. This will prevent you from picking at your meal and eating more than you need while you wait for the others to finish their meal.

Warning: avoid buffets when possible. It's easy to be tempted to overeat to try to get your money's worth.

HEALTH COACH TIPS

Drinking water with your meal will not only save you calories and money, but it can also make you feel fuller so you eat less.

If you are eating at a fast food restaurant, stick to the chain's original or traditional burgers or sandwiches. These are usually smaller and have fewer calories than the other items. Ordering the kid's meal instead of an adult meal is also a way to save calories and limit your portion sizes.

Chapter 9: Getting the Family on Board

My parents came for a visit a few times during my weight loss journey and saw me at a 20-pound weight loss and around a loss of 30 pounds. They didn't come back for a visit until after I had lost 50 pounds. The look on their faces was priceless. My parents questioned what I was doing and how I did it. I was happy to tell them it was whole food and exercise. Simply getting my body moving and incorporating a few tricks here and there, like lemon water in the morning and really restricting sugar and simple carbohydrates is what worked. But, I also had underlying food intolerances that were causing health issues, such as my IBS and eczema. I finally had to remove gluten and dairy to really heal, but that's not always the case for everyone.

Every week I meet with clients who express their challenges in getting their spouse or children to go along with their new healthy lifestyle habits. You could take the route of "this is what I made, so you're going to eat it." Some spouses will just be thankful for a hot meal on the table. Or you can try an all-inclusive approach. You can have a family meeting and discuss the importance of eating healthy and how you want to avoid getting sick, overweight and prevent disease down the road or how you want to heal yourself now. You know your family best and which approach will yield the results you desire.

Involving everyone in the family can help get their attention and approval. You could all go to the farmer's market together where you'll find lots of local food to choose from. Let your kids choose one vegetable and one fruit each. They'll love feeling in charge. Watch a food documentary like Forks over Knives or Food Inc. to understand a little more of the politics involved in our food industry. Start small and make a few little changes at a time. One huge overhaul won't work for them or you.

Spend a little time teaching your older children some basic kitchen skills like properly washing vegetables, whisking, folding, cracking eggs, smashing garlic, knife skills and so on. This gives everyone a personal role in the process and you'll have better success in the long run.

When I enrolled at the Institute for Integrative Nutrition, I had hundreds of lectures to listen to. My husband listened to several of them while we were on road trips in the car. He found some of them to be quite fascinating and some disturbing. This helped to open his eyes to our not-so-honest food world. Plus, he witnessed my amazing health transformation first-hand and practically got a new wife out of the deal! After I dropped 50 pounds, I had such renewed confidence and energy that he quickly came asking for advice on losing weight himself—which he did! Share in the journey together and see how great you and your spouse can feel. It's really empowering to have someone supporting you through this change.

Extended family gatherings

Family gatherings and holidays can be a bit tougher because you don't have the control you do in your own kitchen. I always bring a large platter of fresh cut vegetables and hummus so I have something to eat that includes a protein and some veggies. And it's okay to let your family know that you don't do that well with certain foods. Share how much better you feel when you eat healthier foods.

Choosing this route will not only be an easier way to explain yourself but an overall better invitation to eating a whole foods diet by being an example of feeling great rather than telling your loved ones how they should eat. Trust me, trying to change loved ones' eating habits is the hardest thing to do. It is much better to walk the path, and let them decide if they want to follow.

Choosy kids

I have two very different children: one will try anything and is adventurous in the kitchen and the other is super choosy and quite willful. I tried to start them out with all kinds of vegetables when they were babies, and it worked for my oldest but not so much for my youngest. As she got older, she became more determined at ruining our dinner time. One night she would eat broccoli without a fight and then another night it was like I was feeding her poison. She still protests to this day with certain foods, but now I know why. It was always about texture. If the broccoli was steamed too much and got the least bit mushy, she didn't like it. So, I modified the way I cooked it. I now steam the broccoli for just a few minutes and then finish it off in a skillet with a little oil to give it a crisp texture. She loves it this way!

Picky or choosy kids can really test your patience when it comes to healthy eating. Some will never touch anything green, some don't like cooked veggies and others won't eat any vegetables at all. It's a struggle all moms know very well in trying to get their kids to eat healthier. Some give up and will feed their children anything just so they have something to eat for the day. The process can really take its toll and lead to a lot of struggles and battles with little ones and even your spouse.

Obviously if you can start your healthy eating journey when your children are infants or even in the womb, that would be ideal. Did you know that a baby's first food does not have to be a commercial infant rice cereal? Many pediatric resources are acknowledging the fact that avocado, banana and sweet potato make great first foods for babies.

Also, starting a child too early on rice cereals can present some problems. If a child's starch-digesting enzymes haven't fully matured, the starchy rice cereals can cause allergies and other problems.

As your children get older and their food desires become more known and their "choosiness" starts to rear its ugly head, the best path to take is one of not audibly calling attention to it. What I mean is, don't label your child as "picky" and tell others that he or she won't eat specific foods. We simply talk about all the wonderful foods we have available to us and what they can do for our bodies. For example, I created superhero names for some foods: Cool Carrots have the power of Super Sight; Leafy Lettuce keeps us Lean and Mean; and my personal favorite, The Kale Krusader, fights disease in a single bite! When you attach a fun name and the specific nutritional power a specific food has, it becomes more than just trying to get your child to eat broccoli. Food becomes fun!

My daughters love to look at Pinterest with me. I let each of my girls go through my boards and pick one recipe that they get to help me make for dinner per week. It helps my "choosy" daughter eat more diverse foods too. Sit down with your children and look over the recipes in this book as well.

Be mindful of what and how you eat in front of your children. Your children will pick up any food habits you have as well. If you dislike most vegetables, your children may learn this behavior too. If you always overeat and finish every bite on your plate (because this is the way you were raised), your children will too. A child is born with the ability to sense when they are full. We need to respect that natural instinct they have and not force a child to finish everything on their plate. As adults, we tend to ignore that signal and eat beyond the constraints of our stomachs!

Learn what works for your choosy eater:

- Put several items of her favorite food on her plate and one item of something new. This can be her "try-it" bite.
- Don't use food as a reward or punishment. We don't want to attach feelings of love or hate toward food.
- Don't negotiate. Example: you don't get dessert because you ate only one bite of broccoli.
- If your children are old enough, involve them in the process of food preparation, even if it's just stirring something. Children get excited when they get to create something and then eat it.
- When possible, offer a few different choices without becoming a short-order cook. Some children, and even adults, just don't like certain foods and may never like them, so it's important to have a couple of options during meal times.
- Get them involved at the grocery store. Older children can read grocery lists, help you find certain vegetables and maybe you can even institute the "new veggie of the week" program. Try a new vegetable in a new way each week. Find fun ways to cook with them.
- Presentation matters. Sometimes food just doesn't look that appealing, but when presented in a fun way, like on a stick, kids will gobble it up!
- Give foods a funny name, like the Green Goblin Smoothie or Shrek Smoothie (for my simple green smoothie formula).
- I'm not a fan of hiding vegetables in foods, but if your child won't eat any of them, go ahead and puree or finely chop them into foods like meatloaf, savory breads or soups.
- Always have fresh, whole fruit and vegetables in plain sight or on a shelf they can reach in the fridge. This way they can grab what they like and you can learn what they gravitate toward.

Dinner-time suggestions:

- Turn off the TV, especially the news. Watching something depressing or violent can disturb your digestion.
- Become fully present with your meal. Take a few deep breaths or say a prayer to bring calmness to your body.
- Don't discuss stressful events or bad grades during dinner.
- Take your time during your meal. Eating quickly can create gastric distress.
- Chew your food till it becomes a liquid in your mouth. This stimulates digestive enzymes to further help break down food.

How to keep little ones busy while you cook your healthy meals

I remember dreading dinner time when I had an infant or young toddler. It was the most stressful time of day for me. Like clockwork, at 6 p.m. every night my daughter would scream for two hours straight with an inconsolable colicky cry. Making a healthy dinner was not in the cards, or so I thought. I wish I had known then what I know now! Meals don't have to be complicated. They can be as simple as a poached piece of fish or pan-fried chicken with some steamed veggies.

Here are some tips to keep your little ones busy while cooking:

- Baby wearing is great for infants while you're cooking. The gentle movement can rock them to sleep.
- Give toddlers a special drawer all to themselves. Let them play with spatulas, whisks, plastic measuring cups and a couple of bowls to pretend to stir in.
- Let them arrange large magnets on the fridge.
- Older toddlers and preschoolers can color at the kitchen table or make placemats.

- Set out some cut up veggies like cucumber slices, red bell pepper slices or baby carrots. Let little ones arrange them on a plate. It's okay if they eat a few too! I find pre-dinner crankiness is often due to hunger, so I don't mind them eating some fresh veggies before dinner.
- Older preschoolers can help set the table, put out napkins, get the condiments and set out cups.
- Getting little ones involved in the cooking process at a young age instills a love for real food. Their appreciation and love will grow even deeper if you can involve them in growing some simple vegetables like lettuce or herbs in a small pot or windowsill.

School-aged children

When children enter school, they are exposed to all kinds of food habits. They may even protest eating certain foods. My children stopped eating anything with nuts or peanut butter at school because they were forced to sit at a different table if they have nuts in their food. This frustrated me because my granola bars and trail mix were easy, go-to foods for lunch boxes. They also determined that their princess-themed lunch boxes weren't cool anymore either.

Nevertheless, I like to make their lunch every day because of the processed foods found in school lunches. I visited the cafeteria one day a few years ago and asked to see the boxes the food came in. It was the same stuff from those large food distributors that all have hydrogenated oils, HFCS, numerous preservatives and almost all of it was frozen. We are fortunate enough to have a few local farms that provide fresh vegetables for our school lunches, but they still slather them in rancid oils and sauces and the kids usually don't eat them.

Stocking your back-to-school pantry with some healthy items can be fun! Involve your kids in letting them pick out some new items.

Back-to-school pantry shopping list:

- Lots of whole fruits
    - Ideas: bananas, organic apples, organic peaches, pears, watermelon slices, organic grapes, organic berries, melon balls/cubes, orange slices and small boxes of organic raisins.
    - Make a fun fruit kebab!
    - Whole fruits provide fiber, potassium, antioxidants and tons of vitamins that they need for fuel during the day. (I suggest the organic option of those fruits listed on the Dirty Dozen).
    - Remember to shop and eat seasonally. Some of these fruits won't be available year-round.
- Trail mix
    - Make your own mix with raw, unsalted nuts, pumpkin seeds, sunflower seeds, raisins, dried cranberries, chopped pitted dates, small amount of dark chocolate chips & dried apricots. (NO M&M's!!)
- Wraps
    - Choose whole grain options to wrap up turkey slices, nitrate-free deli meats, peanut butter and jelly, cream cheese and veggies, chicken salad and tuna salad.
- Whole grain English muffins
    - Make mini-pizzas or slather with a nut butter and jam.
- Organic string cheese
- Newman's Own High Protein Pretzels
- Gluten-free?
    - Buy large lettuce leafs and wrap over creamy chicken salad, tuna salad with lots of crunchy pickles and turkey slices (not deli meat).

- Make extra for dinner.
    - o Leftovers make for a great school lunch. Pack hot items in stainless steel or a thermos to retain their heat. My kids' favorites are homemade chicken strips, leftover spaghetti, soups and ravioli.
- Unsweetened organic apple sauce
- Plain organic yogurt
    - o Place in a blender with berries, kale, nut or sunflower butter and honey. Blend and freeze in a flexible popsicle mold.
- Organic ham and cheese roll ups
- Veggies
    - o Sliced cucumbers with hummus, organic celery with nut butter and raisins, carrots with hummus or homemade ranch dip, kale chips and red and yellow pepper slices with hummus or dip.
- Whole grain crackers
    - o Ak-Mak or multi-seed crackers are good options. (Goldfish don't make the cut)
- Brown rice cakes
- Real popcorn
    - o Avoid popcorn microwaved in a chemical-filled bag.
- Hard-boiled eggs
- Roasted chickpeas with honey & cinnamon
- Whole grain waffles
    - o These are great for after-school snacks topped with a nut butter.
- Reusable bottle of ice cold water
    - o Avoid sugary juices.

Chapter 10: Outside Influences on Food Habits

Social gatherings

Be a food snob. If you don't love it, don't eat it, says American Dietetic Association spokeswoman Melinda Johnson, MS, RD. Scan the buffet for foods you truly treasure and skip the everyday dishes that are available all year long. And don't think it's your responsibility to sample everything on the buffet. Go ahead and indulge in your personal holiday favorites, then find a seat and, slowly and mindfully, savor every mouthful. If it's a pot-luck of sorts, I always bring something to share that's a healthy option, like a vegetable platter and hummus. Eat a protein-based snack before you go, so you don't hover by the buffet line.

Eating well at the office

This is another arena where you don't have much control. There may be the never-empty candy bowl in the lunchroom, the Friday donut-day tradition or the snack machines full of candy and packaged food that have enough chemicals to keep them fresh through eternity. Office parties can send your new healthy habits out the window too—but don't let them. Bring a slow-cooker full of a delicious soup, pulled pork or meatballs with a healthy sauce. How about a large, fresh salad with tons of cut vegetables? Always pack yourself a healthy lunch and protein-filled snacks. Some good options are:

- Trail mix
- Homemade granola bars
- Fresh fruit
- Hard-boiled eggs
- Nitrate-free beef sticks or jerky

- Hummus and cut veggies
- Nut butter packets with a banana
- Raw pumpkin and sunflower seeds

Sports snacks

Most snacks during and after games consist of sugar-laden cookies, bags of chips and colorful sports drinks. Children who play sports for an hour or two in the evenings or on weekends, don't need a sport drink or sugary treat when the game is over. What they do need is water, protein and a complex carbohydrate. Coconut water and a banana can replace lost electrolytes much better than an artificial-ly-colored, sugary sports drink. Will the kids on the team grumble about the lack of chips or cookies? Possibly, but children complain about doing their homework and brushing their teeth!

Here are some good alternatives for team snacks:
- Carrot sticks
- Apple slices or mini apples
- Bunch of grapes
- Half a banana
- Clementines, peeled and halved
- Small boxes of raisins
- Baggies of popcorn

These options are typically cheaper than twelve bags of potato chips and a bunch of juice boxes. Ask the parents to make sure every child has a bottle of water, and maybe you can even provide this list and some other healthy options to get the sugar off the field!

Holiday sweets and treats

Valentine's Day, Easter, Halloween and the entire month of December unfortunately revolve around eating copious amounts of candy, cookies, chocolate and marshmallow crème. But, there are ways to limit your child's exposure to excess amounts of sugar, artificial colors and GMOs. Ask your school or child's teacher to distribute a list of non-food items that can be exchanged in class, like pencils, erasers, temporary tattoos, stickers and magnets. At Halloween, my children go through their buckets of candy and pick out up to ten items that are their favorites. The rest gets recycled in various places, like dentist buy-back programs, stockings for soldiers or the trash. When they were little, we would place the bucket of candy on the front porch for the "Switch Witch" and she would bring a trinket or toy, like a puzzle, in place of the candy. My kids loved that.

For holidays, we just learned to scale back. We no longer make 5 to 6 dozen cookies to have lying around for a week. We make 1 to 2 dozen for ourselves and maybe a couple dozen to give away. I use healthier ingredients in the sweet treats as well.

Birthday parties

It's purely my opinion, but I feel that birthday parties have gotten a little out of hand. There's always pizza, a large cake or cupcakes, juice boxes or soda, ice cream and a candy-filled goody bag. This has been the formula for birthday parties for years and my kids will usually come home with a tummy ache and headache. They are starting to make the connection between what they eat and how it makes them feel, which is shaping their choices! I hosted a birthday party once for my oldest and served homemade sub sandwiches, and one child yelled at me and demanded pizza! I like to make cupcakes (without hydrogenated oils), a healthy salad, pasta dish or sandwiches cut into fun shapes with cookie cutters and serve water or homemade lemonade. Their goody bag is usually a small keepsake relating to the theme of the party, like a crown they decorated for a princess theme or a spa bag for a spa party.

Chapter 11: Sustaining Your New Lifestyle

I will share that when our family started on this journey, it wasn't all rainbows, sunshine and lollipops. It was hard, and sometimes we slipped and ordered a pizza for dinner. But the next day, it was back to planning and making sure we got our vegetables in for the day and we were drinking enough water. It's a delicate balance. Another thing our family did was take a year off from afterschool activities. This may not be possible for those of you with older children who are involved in school sports, but for younger children, it definitely makes sense. I didn't have dance, soccer, girl scouts and chorus practice to get to four nights a week when I was young! I was outside running around with my friends. I worry for the kids (and the moms) who are struggling to make it all fit into their schedules. Dinner has taken a back seat (literally!) to sports, clubs and running errands. Make having dinner together a priority, and you'll be amazed at how wonderfully stress-free your evenings can become!

Our habits define us

Good or bad, these habits that you have cause you to look the way you look, act the way you act and feel the way you feel. Your habits will also dictate who you will become in the coming days, weeks, months and years.

But how do you go about **creating change**? You can read dozens of books on diets and pin hundreds of healthy recipes, but how do you apply these changes to your daily life to make them work for you?

The **key** is to make a change and repeat it over and over and over, thus creating a new habit. For example, say you want to start your day off with a 20-minute exercise routine. Every night you need to set out your workout clothes and shoes. Set your alarm for the appropriate time and get up and do your planned exercise. Make a goal of doing this five times per week. Take only two days off.

Or, maybe you need to get more vegetables into your diet. Create a list of your favorites and look up some fun ways to prepare them. Set a goal of getting one vegetable in every meal, even breakfast. Maybe it's spinach in your morning smoothie or omelet, then a huge chicken salad with cut up cucumbers and red peppers for lunch. For dinner, cook two veggie sides with your protein instead of rice or potatoes. Do this every day (of course, changing up your recipes so you don't get bored).

For most of us, it's **fear** that keeps us from moving forward. The unknown can be a very scary place. I didn't know how to cook several years ago. I was scared to get in the kitchen and create something. Following a recipe was like reading a foreign language. But, here's where it gets interesting. Once I did it the first time, I was elated and proud of myself. I made a delicious dinner. Then I did it again and again and again. Cooking became a habit, and following recipes turned into creating and changing recipes into the way I liked them.

Healthy habits can begin in the same fashion. Start with one. Find a habit that resonates with you. Is it only having one cup of coffee per day instead of three? Or perhaps you want to kick your soda habit? Add in another healthier drink or some flavored water. Focus on one thing at a time. Master it. Then, move on and master another until these habits are hard-wired into your brain as something that comes naturally to you. For me, exercise is my release. It's my thinking and planning time. If I start my day without my "zen" time, then I don't feel as well throughout the day. I don't sleep as soundly either.

To make this new lifestyle work for you, you'll need to do some planning. Think hard about what areas you need to improve upon.

Are you snacking on unhealthy items? If so, you'll need to shop for and keep healthy snacks around you. Prepare lots of cut vegetables for the week. Put a plate of them right in the front of the fridge for easy snacking. Some great options are: nuts, trail mix, fresh apples, clementines, grapes, kiwi, sugar snap peas, sliced cucumber, bell peppers, celery sticks and carrot sticks.

Your holiday gatherings may need an overhaul as well. Make lists of holiday menus and the recipes you may need to adjust. It may be time to retire the green bean casserole slathered in that fatty sauce. Try them blanched and sautéed with some sliced shallots and slivered almonds on top.

Spend about 30 minutes prepping food on the weekend. Here's my to-do list on Sundays:

- Wash and prep vegetables when I get home from shopping.
- Prep homemade hummus for snacking.
- Cut up veggies for meals for the week.
- Make 2 cups of quinoa.
- Make chili or butternut squash soup for lunch.
- Chop up a bag of lettuce to make quick salads.

Cook once, eat twice is my golden rule in the kitchen. Always make more than what you'll eat in one meal setting. You can use the leftovers for lunch or stretch them into a meal for another night.

Chapter 12: The Healthy Home

You've cleaned up your pantry and fridge and you're cooking healthier meals, but something is still missing. Maybe you're still having headaches or not breathing as well as you would like. It's time to investigate the rest of the home. According to the Environmental Protection Agency, we spend 90 percent of our time indoors—at home or in our offices. That indoor air can be polluted two to five times more with volatile organic compounds than outdoor air. We got this way by spritzing, painting and cleaning our way through our homes.

Check out these latest alarming trends that might be caused by an unhealthy home:

- The early onset of puberty is increasing, according to researchers at the University of North Carolina. The onset of menstruation used to be 16, but now it's 11.5 years.
- According to BreastCancer.org, only 10 percent of breast cancer is genetic. What else is playing a role here in the alarming rate of breast cancer? Our environment is contributing to this.
- One in 42 boys have autism.
- Pediatric cancer is on the rise.
- Thyroid disease is on the rise.
- Infertility rates are skyrocketing.
- Cancer from toxic chemicals is rising.

There are so many unregulated chemicals in our air, water and food. Currently, manufacturers don't have to prove that toxic chemicals are safe before they go on the market. The laws governing them haven't been updated since 1976.

There are dozens of health risks in your home beyond the foods you eat. I'm going to take you room-by-room and point out the surprising chemicals lurking in everyday products that we've all become familiar with.

In the kitchen

The plastic kitchen!

Take a look around your kitchen. Make note of the plastic spoons, serving utensils, food storage containers, plastic wraps, tumblers, cups, mixing bowls, baby bottles, water bottles, plastic bags and vinyl flooring. We are surrounded by various forms of plastic. Some of those forms of plastic are dangerous to our health. Flip over a plastic bottle or food container and notice those little chasing arrows that have a number inside. Each of those numbers denotes the type of plastic in that product.

1 is PET or polyethylene terephthalate. Found in water and soda bottles, cooking oil containers and frozen food trays. It will degrade over time but it's safe under normal conditions.

2 is HDPE or high-density polyethylene. Found in opaque containers, milk jugs and detergent bottles; not for use for hot liquids. Safe under normal use.

3 is PVC or polyvinyl chloride. Found in shower curtains, vinyl flooring, meat and cheese wrappers and many more places. Avoid this plastic because it contains highly toxic phthalate plasticizers that leach into food.

4 is LDPE or low-density polyethylene. Found in CD cases, plastic bags and packaging. Generally considered safe.

5 is PP or polypropylene. Found in kitchenware, food containers, bottle caps and some hardier take out containers. This is the safest plastic on the market.

6 is PS or polystyrene. Found in take-out containers, cups and egg cartons (think Styrofoam). Highly toxic, especially when heated.

Consider removing your take-out food from these containers and placing it in your own glass food storage containers when you bring it home. Never heat these plastics in the microwave!

7 Other. All other plastics are placed in this category. Includes polycarbonate, acrylic, nylon, fiberglass and hybrid plastics. Specifically found in baby bottles, Nalgene bottles, food processor bowls, blenders and drinking cups. BPA or bisphenol A is found in polycarbonates, which are hard, transparent and glass-like.

NOTE: Not all plastics contain BPA.

What do I avoid?

Avoid plastics with the numbers 1, 3, 6 and 7. Number 7 plastics are tricky. Some (7s) will say BPA-free, but we can't be sure they don't contain Bisphenol F or S. Read below for more information on Bisphenols.

What is BPA?

Bisphenol A or BPA is known as an endocrine-disrupting synthetic estrogen. BPA was first synthesized back in 1891—over 100 years ago. It was developed to serve as a synthetic form of estrogen and was used as such until stronger and more effective synthetic estrogens took its place. In the 1950s, its use shifted to what we have now—an ingredient in plastics.

As a synthetic estrogen, BPA has the ability to block or mimic natural estrogen in the body, which can disrupt the entire endocrine system; hence, the name "endocrine-disrupting chemical." Because of this, it's also included in a class of chemicals referred to as "obesogens." These are chemicals that are directly linked to the altering of our metabolism in ways that can lead to weight gain and obesity as well as result in insulin resistance and diabetes. Obesogens are chemicals that can also interfere with fat cell growth and production. What this means is that some chemicals in this class can not only increase the number of fat cells we end up with but the size of them as well.

Health problems linked to BPA include heart disease, diabetes, insulin resistance, obesity, asthma, breast cancer, prostate cancer, recurring miscarriages, early onset puberty and reduced sperm count as well as developmental and behavioral issues like hyperactivity, impaired learning and delayed development. That's a long list.

Studies looking at prenatal exposures to BPA have shown a dramatic increase in the amount of reproductive birth defects like hypospadias, a birth defect in boys where the urethra doesn't develop at the head of the penis but rather somewhere along the shaft. It's corrected via surgery immediately after being born, but some studies have shown that this birth defect is actually on the rise in human male babies. Prenatal exposure also shows an increase in breast cancer rates and early onset puberty. Not too surprisingly—because of how ubiquitous BPA is—these and other conditions seen in lab animals are also on the rise in humans: higher rates of breast and testicular cancers, ADHD, birth defects, thyroid disease, infertility and sexual dysfunction. Animal studies have shown that prenatal BPA exposure reduces the number of fat cells in the body; this might sound good, but it programs them to incorporate more fat, resulting in fewer but very large fat cells.

Additionally, bisphenol A has a couple of cousins, bisphenol F and bisphenol S. We don't know much about these guys, and likely we will not find it labeled on products we use. I lump them all in the "use with caution" category.

What degrades plastic?

Plastic is made from crude oil and natural gas and linked into flexible chains or polymers. Then, in the final stages of processing, manufacturers add more chemicals to color it as well as add texture, shape and flexibility. These additives can leach out under certain conditions. Heating, microwaving, dishwasher detergents, scrubbing and hot, oily foods can all degrade the plastic and cause dangerous chemicals to leach out.

Heat. Hot foods, high-temperature dishwashers, microwaves

Oil. Oil from cooking oils, citrus oils, fatty foods

Acidity. Tomatoes, citrus

Abrasion. Abrasion from sponges, cleaning brushes, detergents, dishwashers

Time. Time degrades all plastics

HEALTH COACH TIPS

Never use plastic in the microwave, even those that say "microwave-safe." Don't put them in the dishwasher. Use a soft sponge to clean your plastic items, especially those made from polycarbonate, like your food processor bowl or Vitamix blender container. If they get a little foggy, make a paste with water and baking soda to remove the film.

Food storage

Ever notice a tinge of orange lining the inside on some of your plastic food storage containers? I have a few of these that I like to show my clients in workshops. The oil, acidity and abrasion from trying to clean it has caused degradation of the container. Your tomato sauce has migrated into the actual plastic container. So if the sauce is *in* the plastic, the plastic is *in* the sauce.

What do I use instead? Use glass containers from brands like Pyrex, Snapware and Rubbermaid. They may still have plastic lids, so the key is to not let your food touch the lids. Remember, don't ever microwave these containers with their lids on.

Drinking cups and glasses

Plastic drinking cups and containers can contain bisphenol A, S or F, which are endocrine disruptors. According to industry experts, 40 million plastic water bottles end up in landfills every day! Most of these are being used in the office, on the road and on vacations when recycling isn't as readily available as in the home. Plastics should be recycled so that less petroleum is consumed.

What do I use instead? Use glass or a stainless steel reusable bottle and stop buying bottled water. You'll save hundreds of dollars per year by using refillable bottles. I also take my refillable stainless bottle with me when I travel. You can fill it up in an airport café after you pass through security.

Cookware

Non-stick cookware is made with a chemical called perfluorooctanoic acid or PFOA. It goes by the brand name, Teflon®. PFOA is an obesogen and suspected hormone-disrupting chemical and is persistent and bioaccumalative. Every molecule of PFOA that has ever been produced is still around and will be for a long time to come because it has a half-life of 3 to 5 years. According to the CDC, 98 percent of the US population has PFOA circulating in their bodies right now. Because PFOA does not break down, it can get recirculated in our bodies. Animal studies link PFOA exposure to:

- hyperactivity
- reproductive toxicity
- hormone disruption
- immune system toxicity
- thyroid disorders
- cancers

How are we exposed to PFOA? You can be exposed by pre-heating non-stick cookware for just 2 to 3 minutes. PFOA is also found in the lining of microwave popcorn bags, ice cream tubs and frozen food packaging. Never preheat a nonstick pan, and throw it away when they become scratched or start flaking.

What do I use instead? Place a priority on replacing cheap, non-stick cookware and bakeware with heirloom-quality alternatives like cast iron, enameled cast iron, ceramic, stoneware, copper and glass. Replace plastic spatulas, spoons and turners, which are apt to melt if kept too close to the heat, with bamboo or stainless steel.

Around the house

We are all scared of getting sick, but did you know that commonly used items around our homes may be making us sicker? The American Medical Association and the Food and Drug Administration have determined that using antibacterial soaps containing Triclosan do not work any better than plain soap and water at preventing the spread of bacteria. Yet, it's still so very prevalent. This chemical is an endocrine disruptor that can disrupt thyroid function.[47, 48]

Antibacterial soaps

The main ingredient in these hand soaps is a pesticide called **Triclosan**. It's also found in:

- toothpaste
- household cleaners
- hand sanitizers
- antibacterial cutting boards
- treated sponges
- shower curtains
- bath accessories

Triclosan can combine with chlorine that's present in your treated municipal tap water. Most municipalities will add chlorine to their water as a disinfectant. The triclosan will actually react with chlorine at normal hand-washing temperatures and create small clouds of chloroform gas; especially harmful to children who are closer to the faucet. Chloroform gas is a central nervous system depressant and a suspected carcinogen. It also travels into our wastewater and causes sex changes in aquatic life.[49, 50, 51]

What do I use instead? Use plain soap and water. Dr. Bronner's mild castile soap can be diluted in a foaming hand soap dispenser (half soap and half water) and you can add essential oils like thyme or lavender to kill germs and add a natural scent. This will last 6 to 8 months, saving you money on hand soaps.

Fragrance (known as phthalates)

Fragrance may be the most common type of chemical in your house. There are 3,163 chemicals now considered "fragrance." Seventy-five percent of the chemicals used in perfumes and fragrances are endocrine disruptors called phthalates. Used in laundry detergents, fabric softeners, dryer sheets, cleaning supplies, disinfectants, air fresheners, deodorizers, shampoos, hair sprays, gels, lotions, sunscreens, soaps, perfumes, powders and scented candles, fragrances are a class of chemicals that may take you extra time and effort to avoid. But it's worth it. The term "fragrance" or "parfum" on personal care product labels can be a cover for hundreds of harmful chemicals known to be carcinogens, endocrine disrupters and reproductive toxicants, even at low levels.

What do I use instead? Opt for fragrance-free or "100 percent natural fragrance" in personal care items. Skip scented candles and room sprays. These items do not "clean" the air, but instead add dangerous chemicals to the air we breathe.[52]

Personal care products

Every day we use an average of fifteen different types of lotions, creams, shampoos, powders and potions. What you put on your skin might be more toxic than what you put in your body. When you take a warm shower, your pores open up and allow whatever you're rubbing on to be absorbed. So if your shampoo and body wash has a skin-drying sulfate, endocrine-disrupting paraben or fragrance, then it's time to make over your personal care products as well. Our skin is our largest organ and protecting it is crucial. You may think that these chemicals can't really get into your system because they are just washed over your skin or rubbed on the top layer. Yet consider how many transdermal or skin patches there are on the market that contain small amounts of pain relievers, anti-nausea medications, nicotine patches and other pharmaceuticals that are delivered via the skin. These tiny amounts of medicines are absorbed through the skin and delivered right into your bloodstream.

Think about all the products in your bathroom right now. You've got hair dyes, shaving creams, face cream, lotions, makeup remover, body wash, conditioners, tanning creams, antiperspirants, perfume, nail polish, hair gels, mousse, teeth whiteners, hair spray, mascara, lipstick, feminine hygiene products and even toilet paper that have chemicals added to them. Think any of those chemicals are getting absorbed into our body?

A study by the Environmental Working Group (EWG) found more than 200 chemicals present in the umbilical cord of newborn babies.[53] They had to have been absorbed by the mother and then sent to the baby in utero. Some of the chemicals found, like DDT, were banned decades ago, yet they persist in our environment.

Even some of the most popular and trusted brands of face creams, cleansers, sunscreens and shampoos contain chemicals that are classified as obesogens and endocrine-disrupting. Since the government does not require safety testing of these products, manufacturers can and use any chemical they want, regardless of the risks. They will listen to their bottom line, though, and you can vote with your dollars by not buying their products. Look out for these chemicals when purchasing personal care products:

- Parabens (methylparaben, propylparaben, butylparaben). Studies have found that parabens can cause skin irritation, allergic reactions, reproductive health problems and cancer, depending on the form of paraben. Public health experts have been particularly concerned about the longer chain parabens—butylparaben, isopropylparaben, isobutylparaben and propylparaben—because studies have shown that they can mimic the hormone estrogen and disrupt normal function of the hormone system.
- Fragrance (phthalates). As discussed above, fragrance can consist of hundreds of various chemical formulations that have been linked to allergies and asthma, infertility, reduced testosterone concentrations and, most worrisome, abnormal development of reproductive system in baby boys. Consider researching

what your favorite perfume is made of. Look for "100% Natural Fragrance" on labels and avoid products that say "parfum" or "fragrance."

- Sulfates. Try to avoid ingredients that start with "PEG" or have an "-eth" in the middle (e.g., sodium laureth sulfate).

Avoid these ingredients as well:
- Propylene glycol
- Aluminum chlorohydrate (found in antiperspirants)
- DMDM hydantoin
- Imidazolidinyl urea
- Methylchloroisothiazolinone
- Methylisothiazolinone
- Triclosan
- Triclocarban
- Triethanolamine (or "TEA")
- 2-Bromo-2-Nitropropane-1,3 Diol
- BHA
- Boric acid and sodium borate
- DMDM Hydantoin
- Oxybenzone (Found in nearly every chemical sunscreen. EWG recommends that consumers avoid this chemical because it can penetrate the skin, cause allergic skin reactions and may disrupt hormones.[54])
- Retinyl Palmitate (found in sunscreen)
- Octinoxate (found in sunscreen)
- Homosalate (found in sunscreen)
- Octisalate (found in sunscreen)
- Octocrylene (found in sunscreen)

> ## *HEALTH COACH TIP*
>
> Look for mineral-based sunscreens that contain zinc oxide, titanium dioxide and avobenzone. Some good brands include Badger, Babyganics, California Baby, Beauty Counter and The Honest Company.

Baby care products

I was shocked to find so many chemicals in common baby care items as well. Name brand baby wipes and diaper cream contained endocrine-disrupting parabens, fragrance and preservatives. Even delicate baby shampoos and lotions contained quaternium-15—a preservative that acts as a formaldehyde releaser and is known to cause cancer.[55] Make sure you read EVERY label and choose only those products that are pure and safe.

Cleaning indoor air

Indoor air pollution can be worse for those living in a large city. Pollutants such as candles, sofas with stain guard and flame-retardants, new carpet, dust, pet dander, chemicals from cleaners, PFOA from nonstick cookware and even dirty air filters can pollute the air in our homes. Luckily, there are certain houseplants that can filter out these common volatile organic compounds (VOCs). You don't even have to have a green thumb to grow a few of these.

Aloe. This easy-to-grow, sun-loving succulent helps clear formaldehyde and benzene, which can be a byproduct of chemical-based cleaners, paints and more. Aloe is a smart choice for a sunny kitchen window. Beyond its air-clearing abilities, the gel inside an aloe plant can help heal cuts and burns.

Spider plant. Even if you tend to neglect houseplants, you'll have a hard time killing this resilient plant. With lots of rich foliage and tiny white flowers, the spider plant battles benzene, formaldehyde, carbon monoxide and xylene, a solvent used in leather and rubber.

Gerber daisy. This bright, flowering plant is effective at removing trichloroethylene, which you may bring home with your dry cleaning. It's also good for filtering out benzene, which is commonly found in glue, paint, plastics and detergent. One in your bedroom, basement or laundry room would be nice, but it does require lots of light.

Snake plant. Also known as mother-in-law's tongue, this plant is one of the best for filtering out formaldehyde, which is common in cleaning products, toilet paper, tissues and personal care products. Put one in your bathroom; it'll thrive in the steamy humid conditions while helping filter out air pollutants.

Ficus. Place this pretty tall plant in your living room to help filter out pollutants that typically accompany carpeting and furniture such as formaldehyde, benzene and trichloroethylene. Caring for a ficus can be tricky, but once you get the watering and light conditions right, they will last a long time.

Bamboo palm. Also known as the reed palm, this small plant thrives in shady indoor spaces. It tops the list of best plants for filtering out both benzene and trichloroethylene. They're also a good choice for placing around furniture that could be off-gassing formaldehyde.

The laundry room

Consider how many fragrances and chemicals we come into contact with when doing the laundry: the clothes we drape around us, the towels we dry our bodies with, the baby blankets we swaddle our newborns in, the sheets we slip under each night. Laundry detergents and fabric softeners leave behind chemical residues that touch our skin day and night. We are literally bathed in chemical fragrances 24 hours a day!

Laundry detergents

Some of the most popular detergents on the market scored an "F" on EWG's Guide to Healthy Cleaning. Those with added fabric softeners, fragrance and stain-fighting formulas contained the most health-damaging chemicals. They showed a high concern for developmental and reproductive toxicity as well as asthma and respiratory concerns.

You won't find a list of the ingredients on the label either. You have to comb through a series of websites to get to them. I found it intriguing that one name brand detergent listed this statement on their parent company website: "this product contains enzymes, so repeated exposure to the powder may result in sensitization and transient 'hay-fever like' symptoms. The product also contains sodium percarbonate, which is irritating to the mucous lining of the nose, throat and eyes. Additionally, could cause asthma-like symptoms to occur."

What do I use instead? Check your current detergent against the vast database on the EWG website. They provide ratings for over 680 laundry products. They also give a list of those that are safer to use.

Dryer sheets or fabric softeners

Dryer sheets or fabric softeners contain numerous chemicals that alter the fabric of our clothing. They impart a waxy substance that feels soft, but it's not. It's wax. They linger and persist forever. Of the 171 fabric softeners tested by the Environmental Working Group, 83.33 percent of them received a "D" or "F" rating because of their pernicious chemicals and lingering chemical fragrances. Many of these compounds are solvents that directly affect the nervous system and endocrine system and can contribute to the development of chronic illness. Some people may experience a rash or hive from exposure, but most won't see an immediate reaction or ill effect from laundry chemicals, which makes it impossible for them to realize the impact on their health in the long term. Please be careful when considering purchasing a fabric softener or dryer sheets. Twenty-five or more volatile organic compounds are emitted from your dryer with each load when using dryer sheets.

In particular, avoid any synthetic formulas that include these chemicals:

- **Benzyl acetate, chloroform, dichlorobenzene and limonene:** known carcinogens (limonene also irritates eyes and skin).
- **Benzyl alcohol, camphor and biodegradable cationic softeners:** accumulate in the body and cause symptoms ranging from confusion to serious damage to the nervous system.
- **Ethanol and Ethyl Acetate:** two chemicals listed on the Environmental Protection Agency's "hazardous waste" list.
- **Alpha terpineol, pentane and linalool:** cause central nervous system damage, reduced spontaneous motor activity and respiratory issues. Pentane can even cause loss of consciousness and is extremely harmful if inhaled.

What do I use instead? Use wool dryer balls instead of fabric sheets. I like to add a drop of pure Lavender essential oil on my wool dryer balls. You can also add a tablespoon of white vinegar to the rinse cycle, which adds softness and reduces static.

Household cleaners

I find it ironic that we actually contaminate the air inside our home when we "clean" it. Mixing household cleaners, especially ammonia with bleach, can produce a deadly cocktail of gases. Ammonia can trigger asthmatic attacks and cause lung cells to dissolve. Mixing bleach with a phosphate cleaner will release chlorine gas—also known as mustard gas—as well as hypochlorous acid. Twenty-five states and the District of Columbia have imposed a variety of restrictions or bans on laundry and dishwasher detergents and other cleaning supplies containing phosphates in order to reduce pollution from wastewater. Phosphorus pollution triggers algal blooms that can be toxic to people, harmful to aquatic life and costly to remove from drinking water sources.

Consider this fact: Bleach is involved in more household poisonings than any other chemical.

What do I use instead? One part white distilled vinegar to nine parts water will kill 90 percent of bacteria and many spores. You can buy a gallon under two dollars and make more than 10 gallons of cleaning solution with that. I like Branch Basics brand cleaner, which contains plant-based enzymes and can clean every surface of your home. Other natural supplies to have on hand include baking soda and pure essential oils that have antibacterial properties like thyme, oregano, tea tree oil and cinnamon.

Oven cleaners

These contain dangerous chemicals known to cause cancer, restrict breathing and cause skin rashes. Some of the most popular brands in the U.S. are banned in the European Union.

What do I use instead? Sprinkle baking soda liberally over the bottom of your oven, spray with water, wait 8 hours, scrape and wipe clean.

Dry cleaning

Dry cleaning is actually a wet process wherein solvents are used to remove dirt and stains. This solvent is called Perchloroethylene (PERC), and it is a central nervous system depressant that can enter the body through the lungs and skin. Long-term exposure can cause kidney and liver damage and has been proven in laboratories to cause cancer in animals. In 1990, the United States Congress listed PERC as a hazardous air pollutant in subsection (b) of Section 112 of the federal Clean Air Act.

The International Agency for Research on Cancer (IARC) has classified PERC in Group 2A as a probable human carcinogen. In addition to the cancer effects, acute toxic effects resulting from short term exposure to high levels of PERC may include headaches, dizziness and rapid heartbeat as well as irritation or burns on the skin, eyes or respiratory tract. The good news is that California and a few other states have ordered that PERC be phased out by the year 2023.[56]

What do I use instead? Look to see if your community has an "eco-friendly" dry cleaner who uses paraffin-based cleaning agents or, even better, liquid CO_2, an effective, nontoxic method. If you don't have one nearby, air out your dry cleaned items by removing the plastic covers and hanging them in a well-ventilated area like a garage before bringing them inside. Never store your newly dry-cleaned items in your closet with the plastic still on. This concentrates the chemicals and VOCs even longer.

Outside the Home

Driveway sealant

Avoid coal-tar based sealants that contain polycyclic aromatic hydrocarbons. Studies suggest they are carcinogenic, toxic and mutagenic.

What do I use instead? Choose asphalt sealant or gravel.

Weed killers

Researchers have linked pesticides and herbicides to various forms of cancer, including non-Hodgkin's lymphoma. Insecticides have been connected to brain damage in kids. Pesticides and chemical fertilizers kill the health of the soil and create a lawn that allows for little rainwater absorption, which contributes to flooding. Roundup weed killer (which contains 18 percent glyphospate) actually says it's toxic to aquatic life right on the label. What happens when it rains and residues make their way down storm drains?

What do I use instead? Try removing weeds by the root or spray them with undiluted vinegar. Corn gluten prevents dandelions and crab grass from germinating, and it also feeds the grass, making it stronger and more resistant to weeds. Apply to your lawn in early spring.

Pesticides

Pesticides in and around the home are very dangerous and residues can last for months and even up to one year. They have been found to be endocrine disruptors, which can lead to weight gain, interference with the natural hormone systems that regulate metabolism and disturbance of hormone levels. [57]

What do I use instead? Use caulk at pest entry points and natural pest control measures like essential oils and diatomaceous earth, which can be found at home and garden centers.

Chapter 13: Healthy Recipes

Breakfast

SIMPLE GREEN SMOOTHIE

Green smoothies are very trendy right now, but they serve a great purpose: to get nutrients in you in a quick and healthy manner! There's a simple formula to making green smoothies.

2 cups leafy greens (spinach, Swiss chard, romaine or baby kale)

2 cups water or almond/coconut milk

1 banana or pitted date (this is your sweetener)

1 cup of fresh or frozen fruit

1. Blend greens and water.

2. Add fruit and banana and blend again.

Tip: If you have a high-powered blender, you can add all items at once and blend.

Tip: Frozen fruit or a frozen banana makes it creamy and cold. Berries can make it purple or pink and pineapple makes it bright green, which can be fun for kids. Give it a fun name, like the Pink Princess Smoothie or Green Goblin Smoothie!

Serves 2.

SUPERFOOD SMOOTHIE

2 cups leafy greens (spinach, Swiss chard, romaine or baby kale)

2 cups water, coconut water or almond/coconut milk

1 banana or pitted date (this is your sweetener)

1 cup of fresh or frozen fruit

Superfood Boosts

1 tablespoon chia seeds

1 tablespoon ground flax seeds

1 teaspoon maca powder

1 tablespoon raw cacao

½ avocado, 1 tablespoon nut butter, 1 tablespoon coconut oil or
coconut manna (choose 1 fat)

Dash cinnamon

1. Blend greens and water.
2. Add fruit and banana and blend again.

Tip: If you have a high-powered blender, you can add all items at once and blend.

Tip: You can choose a few of these or all for your smoothie. Play around with different ingredients to find a combination you enjoy.

Serves 2.

5-Minute Omelet

2 farm-fresh eggs

Handful of spinach or leftover vegetables from dinner

Sea Salt and Pepper

1. Crack eggs in a bowl and scramble.
2. Heat a small 8-inch skillet with a teaspoon of coconut or olive oil.
3. Add the eggs and then place the spinach or vegetables on top of the eggs.
4. Crack fresh salt and pepper on the eggs.
5. Swirl the pan around to spread the egg mixture around for even cooking.
6. Let set for 2–3 minutes.
7. Shake the pan to see if it's ready to be flipped. If it sticks, it's not ready yet.
8. Flip the omelette over and cook 1–2 minutes on other side.
9. Slide out onto and plate and fold over the eggs.
10. Serve with fresh salsa and half an avocado, diced.

Serves 1.

1-Minute Mug Muffin

¼ cup ground flax seeds
½ teaspoon aluminum-free baking powder
Heavy dash of cinnamon
Dash of vanilla extract
1 teaspoon chia seeds (optional)
Handful of chopped walnuts or pecans
1 teaspoon olive oil or avocado oil
1 egg
Handful of fresh berries
1 tablespoon honey or maple syrup

1. Crack 1 egg into a large coffee cup and beat.
2. Add the remaining ingredients and gently stir.
3. Heat on a normal temperature in a microwave for 1 minute.
4. Enjoy right out of the mug or invert onto a plate.

Serves 1.

Classic Pancakes

1 ½ cups unbleached flour
3 tablespoons sugar (sucanat or pure cane sugar)
1 tablespoon aluminum-free baking powder
½ teaspoon sea salt
1 ¼ cups 2 percent milk, organic preferably
½ stick melted butter or ghee
2 eggs
Dash of vanilla extract
Heavy dash of cinnamon
Add-ins: blueberries, banana slices, mini chocolate chips

1. In one bowl, whisk together flour, sugar, cinnamon, baking powder and salt.

2. In another bowl, whisk milk, butter, eggs and vanilla, and pour into the flour mixture.
3. Ladle ¼ cupfuls onto a hot, buttered flat-top grill pan or skillet.
4. Put your favorite add-ins onto the pancake as it cooks.
5. Cook until bubbles appear and then flip to continue cooking on the other side.
6. Serve with real maple syrup.

Tip: To ease you into a whole wheat version, use ¾ cup each all-purpose and whole wheat flour.

Serves 4.

CHIA PUDDING WITH PEANUT BUTTER

1 ½ cups coconut milk (full-fat from a can)
¼ cup chia seeds
1 tablespoon sweetener of your choice (raw honey or real maple syrup)
1 banana
½ cup walnuts
4 tablespoons peanut butter (unsweetened)
Handful blueberries or raspberries (fresh or frozen)

1. Mix the coconut milk and honey in a mason jar to combine.
2. Add the chia seeds, put the lid on the jar and shake to combine.
3. Place it in the fridge overnight.
4. The next morning, layer your pudding with chia pudding, 1 tablespoon peanut butter, a few banana slices, a few walnuts and berries, more chia pudding, and so on.

Tip: This is a great on-the-go meal.

Serves 1-2.

HOMEMADE GRANOLA

   3 cups of quick cooking oats (not the big flat rolled oats)
   1 cup of mixed raw, unsalted nuts (I like almonds, cashews, walnuts and brazil nuts)
   ¼ cup raw pumpkin seeds
   ¼ cup raw, unsalted sunflower seeds
   1 tablespoon chia seeds
   6 tablespoons unrefined coconut oil
   6 tablespoons raw local honey
   1 heaping teaspoon cinnamon
   Pinch of ginger
   Pinch of Celtic sea salt
   1 teaspoon almond extract (okay to substitute with vanilla extract)
   Add-ins: dried tart cherries, raisins, chocolate chips or dried fruit

1. Preheat oven to 250 degrees.
2. Put nuts in a food processor and pulse till they are pebbles. Don't pulse too much; you don't want a flour texture. Big nutty chunks are okay.
3. Add oats and pulse two more times.
4. Place oats, nuts, seeds, cinnamon, ginger, sea salt and chia seeds into a big bowl and stir to combine.
5. In a small saucepan, heat the coconut oil and honey over very low heat until melted and combined, about 45 seconds.
6. Add the almond extract.
7. Pour this over the oat mixture. Stir to coat.
8. Dump onto a parchment paper-lined, rimmed cookie sheet. (Foil is okay to use in a pinch.)
9. Bake at 250° for 55 minutes. Check it about 30 minutes through and use a spatula to turn. Pull it out and let it cool.

10. Add dried fruit, raisins or other mix-ins.

Note: I don't like the texture of the dried fruit when baked. They get too dry, so I add them afterward.

Tip: Store in glass mason jars or plastic bags. Store in an air-tight container for up to two weeks.

Makes 2 quarts.

LOADED OATMEAL

4 cups filtered water
2 cups rolled oats
Dash of cinnamon
2 tablespoons of apple cider vinegar

1. Mix together the above ingredients in your pot and leave on the countertop at room temperature overnight.
2. Next morning: bring to boil, remove from heat and let sit covered for 10 minutes.
3. Add in the following optional toppings: Fresh berries, chopped nuts, sliced banana, swirl of nut butter, chia seeds, flax seeds, raisins, scoop of protein powder or diced apples.

Eggs 4 Ways

SWEET POTATO HASH

1. Dice 1–2 small sweet potatoes.
2. Fry in a skillet with a tablespoon of coconut oil or ghee.
3. Beat 2 large eggs and pour over potatoes.
4. Scramble the eggs throughout the hash.
5. Season with salt and pepper. Serves 2.

Eggs in a Basket

1. Cut out the center of a slice of whole grain bread.
2. Melt ghee in a skillet over medium heat.
3. Place the bread in the pan and crack an egg into the center.
4. Toast the cutout portion.
5. Season the egg with salt and pepper.
6. When the egg is mostly set, flip over and cook for another minute. Serves 1.

Eggs Poached over Greens

1. Chop a small bunch of curly leaf kale.
2. Heat coconut oil in a skillet and place greens inside.
3. Add a splash of chicken stock or water.
4. Salt and pepper and cover for 3 to 5 minutes.
5. Stir occasionally and turn off heat when tender.
6. Fill a large, deep-sided skillet with water and heat to almost a boil.
7. Swirl the water with a spoon and crack 2 eggs into the simmering water.
8. For medium poached eggs, usually 5 minutes is all you need.
9. Test the yolk with the back of a spoon to see if it "gives."
10. Remove with a slotted spoon when done to your liking.
11. Set atop braised kale greens. Serves 2.

Quick Frittata

1. Preheat oven to 350 degrees.
2. Use any leftover sausage or beef from a previous meal.
3. Heat 1 tablespoon coconut oil in an oven-safe skillet (like cast iron).
4. Add your meat and heat through.

5. Add any leftover veggies, like diced bell peppers, mushrooms, onions, sun-dried tomatoes or whatever you have on hand.

6. Crack 4 eggs and a couple tablespoons of milk into a bowl and beat.

7. Add egg mixture to the skillet and season with salt and pepper.

8. Cook for 3–5 minutes or until the bottom is set. Add cheese if desired.

9. Place into the hot oven for 10–15 minutes. You can also put the oven on broil for the last 2 minutes to brown the top.

10. Remove from the oven and slide out onto a plate. Slice like a pizza. Serves 2-3.

WARM WINTER SMOOTHIE

1 ½ cups coconut or almond milk
1 tablespoon nut butter (I like cashew butter)
1 tablespoon chia seeds
1 teaspoon maca powder
1 teaspoon raw cacao (or cocoa powder)
1 tablespoon raw honey or several drops of liquid Stevia
Splash of pure vanilla extract
1 teaspoon coconut oil
½ teaspoon cinnamon
Dash of ginger, nutmeg, turmeric, cardamom, sea salt

1. Put all of the ingredients into a saucepan and warm over low heat. You don't want it to come to a bubble because high heat destroys the nutritional properties of the honey and cacao.

2. Gently stir to combine everything.

3. Pour into a blender and whip till frothy.

4. Pour into a mug, sprinkle with cinnamon or extra chia seeds and enjoy on a cold day!

Serves 1.

FAT-BURNING CHOCOLATE BREAKFAST SMOOTHIE

½ avocado

5–6 Brazil nuts

1 tablespoon chia seeds

1 tablespoon raw pumpkin seeds

1 tablespoon sunflower seeds

½ teaspoon Maca powder

1 tablespoon Raw Cacao

Pinch of cinnamon

Handful blueberries or other seasonal berry

1 tablespoon MCT Oil or unrefined coconut oil (melted)

NuNaturals Stevia drops (5–6 drops or to taste)

½ cup to 1 cup filtered water

5–6 ice cubes

1. Place all ingredients into a high-powered blender.
2. Blend.

Tip: Enjoy right away, but you can make the night before, you will need to give it a quick whirl in the morning to incorporate any ingredients that have settled.

Serves 1.

YOGURT PARFAIT

Add 6 oz. Greek yogurt

½ cup fruit

2 tablespoons granola

drizzle of honey

Serves 1.

More breakfast ideas

- Almond butter on top of a sliced banana
- Mashed Avocado on toast

- Hard-boiled eggs
- Eggs/bean/cheese wrap
- Buckwheat frozen waffles with nut butter and fruit

Lunch Recipes

THE LUNCH BOWL

Over the weekend or when you have extra time, make a large batch of brown rice or quinoa. I will usually make 2–3 cups on Sunday to have for the week.

The Lunch Bowl is a leftover mish-mash. Place your base of seasoned rice or quinoa on the bottom of the bowl. Then add leftover or fresh veggies and leftover protein from dinner or a can of tuna or chick peas. You can add nuts, sunflower or pumpkin seeds as well as avocado and a simple dressing of olive oil and balsamic vinegar.

25-MINUTE BUTTERNUT SQUASH SOUP

  1 onion, peeled and chopped into quarters
  1 large apple, peeled, quartered and core removed
  2–3 cups chicken stock (can use water or vegetable or turkey
    stock)
  1 large butternut squash, peeled and seeded, cut into 1-inch
    cubes
  Pinch of cinnamon
  Dash of nutmeg, ground ginger, dried sage
  1 teaspoon dried thyme
  1–2 teaspoon sea salt, ground black pepper
  2 tablespoons dry-roasted pumpkin seeds, optional
  2 tablespoons grass-fed butter

1. In a soup pot, add all ingredients, except butter and pumpkin
   seeds.

2. Add enough chicken stock to come just under the top of the squash. If you have too much, your soup will be too watery and not enough will make it too thick.

3. Bring to a boil.

4. Cover and cook on medium heat 20 minutes or until the veggies are soft.

5. You can then either puree with an immersion or stick blender or put into a food processor or blender and puree till smooth. If using a normal blender, be sure to place a kitchen towel over the top to avoid the hot soup from spraying out.

6. Add 2 tablespoons grass-fed butter and swirl into the warm soup.

7. Pour into bowls and garnish with toasted pumpkin seeds, or you can try cooked, crumbled bacon or sour cream or a drizzle of coconut milk.

Makes 1 ½ quarts.

Power Salad & Homemade Dressings

POWER SALAD LUNCH

Each day, create your filling salad. Here's how . . .

Start with lettuce	2 cups, any variety or mix.	spinach, arugula, spring mix
Add unlimited veggies	Go for at least a one-cup mix of options.	raw tomatoes, cucumbers, onions, bell peppers, shredded carrots, cabbage, sugar snap peas, broccoli, etc.
Add a filling protein	Choose one option. *Want to add two? A half-portion of each is fine!	3-ounce grilled chicken 3-ounce tuna or salmon 2 sliced hard-cooked omega-3 eggs ¾ cup shelled, organic edamame 2/3 cup chickpeas ½ cup cooked quinoa.

Add a flat-belly bonus	Choose one option. *Want to add two? A half portion of each is fine!	¼ cup shredded cheese 3 tablespoons sliced almonds or other nuts 20 olives 2 tablespoons sunflower seeds 2 tablespoons dried fruit ½ avocado can be added each time
Toss with homemade dressing	Choose one option.	1 ½ teaspoon olive oil plus red wine vinegar and herbs to taste 2 tablespoons Newman's Own Red Wine Vinegar & Olive Oil Lite Dressing

Homemade salad dressings are very easy to make. They're basically 60 percent oil (olive oil, nut oil or flax oil), 30 percent acidic medium (balsamic, lemon juice, apple cider vinegar, red wine or rice vinegar) and 10 percent spices, herbs and flavors.

HOMEMADE POPPYSEED DRESSING

½ cup avocado oil (or any nut oil; olive oil works too)
3 tablespoons apple cider vinegar
2 tablespoons raw honey
1 tablespoon poppy seeds
Pinch of ground dry mustard (optional)
Celtic sea salt and pepper

Whisk all ingredients together until combined or pour into a mason jar and shake! Let the kids help with this part!

Serves 4.

BALSAMIC VINAIGRETTE

6 tablespoons extra virgin olive oil
3 tablespoons balsamic vinegar
1 teaspoon Dijon mustard
1 minced garlic clove
Juice of ½ lemon
Pinch of Celtic sea salt and pepper

Pour into a mason jar and shake or whisk in a glass bowl.

Tip: Store for 2 days in the fridge. It will separate, so shake it before each use.

Serves 4–6.

HOMEMADE RANCH

    ½ cup buttermilk
    ¼ cup mayonnaise
    ½ tablespoon chopped parsley
    ½ tablespoon chopped chives
    1 tablespoon apple cider vinegar
    ¼ teaspoon sea salt
    Pinch of onion powder and garlic powder

1. Whisk together ingredients.
2. Chill for 30 minutes before serving.

Tip: You can substitute plain yogurt for the mayonnaise and 2 percent milk in place of the buttermilk.

Serves 4-6.

AVOCADO TAHINI DRESSING

    1 ripe avocado
    1 tablespoon tahini
    3 tablespoons balsamic vinegar
    1 tablespoon extra virgin olive oil
    1 cup water
    1 small clove garlic, chopped

Place the ingredients in a high-speed blender and mix well.

Tip: Store in the fridge for up to 2 days.

Serves 4.

THOUSAND ISLAND DRESSING

½ cup mayonnaise

⅓ cup sweet chili sauce

2 tablespoons sweet pickle relish

1 tablespoon chopped chives

1 hard-boiled egg, finely minced

Juice of ½ lemon

1. Whisk all ingredients.
2. Place in the fridge for 15 minutes to chill.

Serves 4.

PORTABELLA MUSHROOM PIZZA

2 portobello mushroom sliders, stems removed

3–4 basil leaves or ¼ teaspoon dried basil

3–4 spinach leaves

4 tablespoons marinara sauce

2 tablespoons shredded cheese

Sea salt and pepper

1. With a damp cloth or paper towel, remove the dirt from the mushroom.
2. Place 2 sliders on a small baking tray, gill side up.
3. Divide basil and spinach leaves on top of each mushroom.
4. Season with salt and pepper.
5. Spoon marinara sauce on top.
6. Sprinkle with shredded cheese.
7. Place into a 350-degree oven for 10 to 15 minutes.

Serves 1.

Tip: You can also do this in a toaster oven for 10 to 15 minutes on 350 degrees.

SWISS CHARD WRAPS

2 large Swiss chard leaves
½ avocado, mashed
1 teaspoon Dijon mustard
2–3 slices sliced turkey breast or uncured ham
Handful chopped lettuce, sliced carrots or cucumber

1. Spread mashed avocado and Dijon on chard leaves.
2. Layer your turkey or ham and place veggies on top.
3. Roll each leaf like a cigar and cut diagonally.

Tip: Swiss chard or large lettuce leaves make a great gluten-free sandwich. Plus, it's a great way to get some extra veggies into your diet.

QUINOA TABBOULEH

Quinoa is a complete protein and great for energy. I love the nutty crunch! Very simple and quick.

1 cup cooked quinoa
¼ cup cucumber, diced
½ small tomato, diced
Handful chopped herbs, like cilantro, mint, basil or parsley
Juice of ½ lemon
Extra virgin olive oil
Sea salt and pepper
Feta cheese (optional)

1. Cook 1 cup of quinoa according to package directions and chill for 20 minutes.
2. When cool, add diced cucumber, tomato and chopped herbs.
3. Squeeze the juice of ½ lemon and a drizzle of olive oil over your bowl.

4. Season with Celtic sea salt and pepper.
5. Optional: add feta cheese crumbles.

Caprese Salad

This is one of my all-time favorite appetizers that I can enjoy right from my summer garden.

2 beefsteak or large Roma tomatoes
1 small ball of buffalo mozzarella, sliced
Handful of basil leaves
Drizzle of Balsamic vinegar & Extra Virgin Olive Oil
Sea salt & black pepper

1. Cut a large beefsteak or Roma tomato into slices.
2. Add a slice of buffalo mozzarella and a few basil leaves on top of tomato slices.
3. Drizzle with a good, aged Balsamic vinegar and extra virgin olive oil.
4. Sprinkle with sea salt and pepper.
   Serves 4.

Soups

Summer Gazpacho

3–4 Roma tomatoes
1 sweet or vidalia onion
1 small red onion
1 green bell pepper
1 red bell pepper
2 cucumbers
1–2 garlic cloves, minced
2 tablespoons fresh basil

2 tablespoons fresh cilantro
1 seeded, diced jalapeno
4 cups tomato juice (check the label to make sure it's healthy)
2 tablespoons lemon juice
2 tablespoons balsamic vinegar
Dash of hot pepper sauce
¼ cup extra virgin olive oil
Celtic sea salt and fresh ground pepper

1. Bring a large pot of water to boil. Place an "X" on the bottom of your tomatoes with a sharp knife. Drop into boiling water for 30 seconds. Take out and place into a large bowl of cold, icy water. The skin will peel off very easily now.
2. Set out two large bowls. One bowl will be for your toppings, one will be for the items that go into a blender.
3. Dice tomatoes, removing most of the seeds. Place all but one into a large bowl. Save one, small, diced tomato for the toppings bowl.
4. Dice one cucumber small for the toppings bowl, one larger for the blender.
5. Dice the peppers, onions, cilantro and basil. Larger pieces for the blender bowl and the smaller dices for the toppings bowl.
6. In a separate bowl, mix the vinegar, lemon juice, tomato juice, olive oil, salt, pepper and hot sauce with a small whisk.
7. Place the larger cut vegetables, garlic and jalapeno into a blender or Vitamix and pulse for just a few seconds (not too long) to get everything blended.
8. Pour this mixture into your toppings bowl. Then pour the vinegar mixture on top and stir. Adjust your seasonings and let chill for 2 to 3 hours.
9. Serve with a squeeze of lemon juice and more diced cucumber on top.

Serves 6–8.

"Cream of" Soups

BASIC WHITE SAUCE

    3 tablespoons butter or ghee
    3 tablespoons whole wheat flour, white wheat flour or GF flour
    ¼ teaspoon sea salt
    Dash of pepper
    1 ¼ cup liquid, milk or stock

1. Melt butter in saucepan.
2. Stir in flour and seasonings.
3. Cook over medium heat until bubbly.
4. Add liquid slowly, stirring with wire whisk to prevent lumps.
5. Add ¼ teaspoon garlic powder and ¼ teaspoon onion powder.
6. Cook until thick.

Makes 1 cup or 1 can of condensed soup.

TOMATO SOUP

Use jarred tomato juice for the liquid. Add dashes of garlic, onion powder, basil and oregano.

CONDENSED CHICKEN SOUP

Use chicken broth for half the liquid. Add ¼ teaspoon poultry seasoning or sage.

MUSHROOM/CELERY/CHIVE SOUP

Saute ¼ cup chopped mushrooms, celery or chives and 1 tablespoon minced onion in butter before adding flour.

WHITE CHICKEN CHILI

    1 medium onion, finely chopped
    3 tablespoons coconut oil or ghee

1 4-ounce can chopped green chiles

3 tablespoons flour

2 teaspoons cumin

2 cups chicken broth

2 cans great northern beans

1 ½ cups finely chopped, cooked chicken

1. Cook onions in oil until transparent.

2. Add chiles, cumin and flour.

3. Cook and stir for 2 minutes.

4. Add beans and chicken stock.

5. Bring to a boil.

6. Add the cooked chicken and remove from the heat.

7. Toppings: shredded jack cheese, sour cream, fresh salsa, diced avocado.

Serves 4-6.

Slow-Cooker Chicken Enchilada Soup

3–4 organic chicken breasts (cut into tenders) and/or thighs

1 med onion, diced

2 cans Eden Black Beans, rinsed (Eden uses BPA-free can linings)

28-ounce diced tomatoes

10-ounce mild enchilada sauce (I use Frontera brand that has no preservatives)

1 teaspoon cumin, chili powder, sea salt, black pepper

1 teaspoon chopped cilantro

1 quart organic chicken broth

10-ounce bag frozen organic corn

1. Place all ingredients into a 6-quart crock pot and turn on high for 4 hours or low for 6–8 hours.

2. After 3 hours, shred chicken with two forks.

3. Cover pot to remain cooking.

Serves 6–8.

Here's where the fun comes in! Have the kids help with setting up a toppings bar:

    Shredded cheese
    Sour cream
    Chopped cilantro
    Lime wedges
    Crushed tortilla chips or strips
    Avocado slices
    Hot Sauce (if you like it spicy!)

THAI CHICKEN COCONUT SOUP (TOM KHA GAI)

This Thai chicken soup gets its rich flavor from classic Thai ingredients: coconut milk, lemongrass, fresh ginger, lime juice, chili paste, basil and cilantro. Takes only 20 minutes!

    1 can full-fat 14-ounce coconut milk
    14 ounce reduced-sodium chicken broth or homemade stock
    6 fresh ginger slices, 1-inch pieces
    1 stalk fresh lemongrass, 1-inch pieces
    1 pound boned, skinned chicken breast or thighs, 1-inch chunks
    1 cup sliced mushrooms
    1 tablespoon fresh lime juice
    1 tablespoon Thai or Vietnamese fish sauce
    1 teaspoon sugar, sucanat or coconut palm sugar
    1 teaspoon Thai chili paste
    ¼ cup fresh basil leaves
    ¼ cup fresh cilantro

1. In a medium saucepan, combine coconut milk, broth, ginger and lemongrass.

2. Bring to boil over high heat.
3. Add chicken, mushrooms, lime juice, fish sauce, sugar and chili paste.
4. Reduce heat and simmer until chicken is firm and opaque, 5–10 minutes.
5. Discard lemongrass.
6. Garnish servings with basil and cilantro.

Serves 4.

QUICK THAI COCONUT CURRY SOUP

1. Mince 2 small **shallots** in coconut oil.
2. Add 2 tablespoons **green curry paste** and 1 **red bell pepper** cut into small strips.
3. Add 2 cans light **coconut milk** and ¼ cup **stock**.
4. Add leftover cooked **chicken** and top with chopped **cilantro, mint**, squeeze of **lime** juice, **bean sprouts** and diced **scallions**.
Serves 2.

Side Dishes

BRAISED COLLARD GREENS

1 bunch of rinsed collard greens
½ medium onion, diced
1 clove of garlic, minced
Pinch of red pepper flakes (optional)
Sea salt and pepper
1 tablespoon bacon grease or lard
2–3 tablespoons homemade chicken stock or water

1. Prepare the collards green leaves by laying them flat, rolling into a cigar and cutting down the line. Then, turn your cutting board

and cut along the other direction till you get a small rough chop.

2. Heat the lard in a large skillet or braising pan over medium heat.

3. Add the diced onion and cook until soft.

4. Add the minced garlic and stir for 10 seconds.

5. Add the collards and stir to coat the leaves.

6. Add seasonings.

7. Add the stock or water and cover with a lid to wilt the leaves, about 10–12 minutes.

8. Remove the lid and allow the water to cook off for about 1–2 minutes. Serve immediately.

Serves 4.

SAUTEED KALE

1 bunch of fresh, curly leaf kale
1 clove of garlic, minced
Pinch of red pepper flakes (optional)
Sea salt and pepper
1 tablespoon coconut oil
2–3 tablespoons homemade chicken stock or water

1. Heat the oil in a skillet over medium heat.

2. Add the minced garlic and stir for 10 seconds.

3. Add the kale and stir to coat the leaves.

4. Add seasonings.

5. Add the stock or water and cover with a lid to wilt the leaves, about 3–4 minutes.

6. Remove the lid and allow the water to cook off for about 1–2 minutes.

7. Serve immediately.

Serves 4.

Tip: Use any leftovers to fill an omelet for breakfast.

BAKED ACORN SQUASH

1. Cut **squash** into chunks.
2. Drizzle **olive oil**, **sea salt** and **pepper** over them.
3. Cover with foil and bake at 375 degrees for 45–50 min.
4. Remove foil and finish cooking for 10–15 more minutes.
   Serves 4.

QUINOA

1. Rinse 1 cup of **quinoa** in a fine mesh strainer under cool water.
2. Place in a saucepan with 2 cups of water and a pinch of **sea salt**.
3. Turn on high and bring to a boil.
4. Cover and reduce to low for 15 min.
5. Fluff with a fork and serve as a side dish.
   Tip: We like ours with a sprinkle of feta cheese.
   Makes 2 cups.

SPAGHETTI SQUASH

    1 spaghetti squash
    2 tablespoons grass-fed butter
    Sea salt & black pepper

1. Preheat oven to 425 degrees.
2. Cut squash in half and place in a 13 x 9 glass dish.
3. Add 2 tablespoons butter and salt and pepper to both halves.
4. Flip over, cut side down.
5. Bake for 45 minutes at 425 degrees.
6. When done, scrape the sides down with a fork into long strands.
7. Scoop out on plates and sprinkle with a little more salt and pepper.

Tip: For a sweeter version, sprinkle with cinnamon and brown sugar instead.

Serves 4.

CAULIFLOWER RICE

1 small head cauliflower, cut into florets
1 tablespoon coconut oil, olive oil or butter/ghee
Splash of chicken stock
Sea salt and pepper

1. Place the raw cauliflower into a food processor and pulse until it has a grainy rice-like consistency. Season with sea salt and freshly ground black pepper.
2. Sauté the cauliflower in a pan with oil and add any additional seasonings desired (garlic, ginger, curry, etc) until warm and soft.
3. You can add a splash of chicken stock and cover to steam as well.
4. Serve.

Tip: *If using olive oil, do not bring to a sizzle.

Serves 4.

MASHED CAULIFLOWER

1 head cauliflower
2 cloves garlic
2 tablespoons pastured butter
Sea salt and pepper

1. Chop up the head of cauliflower (florets and stem) and slice the garlic.
2. Steam the cauliflower and garlic for about 10 minutes, or until the cauliflower is very tender.
3. Transfer the cauliflower and garlic to a food processor and add the butter.

4. Process until smooth and creamy. You may add some coconut milk and/or water.

5. Season to taste with salt and pepper and serve.

Serves 4.

RED POTATO SALAD

    1 ½ pound small red-skinned or new potatoes

    3 ½ tablespoons apple cider vinegar

    2 teaspoon Dijon mustard

    2 tablespoons extra virgin olive oil

    2 hard-boiled eggs, peeled and cut into pieces

    1 green onion, finely diced

    Sea salt and pepper

1. Cook potatoes in boiling salted water until fork-tender, about 12 minutes. Drain water.

2. When potatoes are cool enough to handle, cut into quarters.

3. Whisk vinegar and mustard together in a large bowl.

4. Add in oil in a small stream while whisking until well combined.

5. Add green onions.

6. Add warm potatoes and combine with dressing.

7. Add eggs and season with salt and pepper.

Makes 4 cups.

SPRING VEGETABLE MEDLEY

    1 cup of fresh peas

    1 bunch of asparagus

    ½ red onion, sliced

    1 kohlrabi, cut into sticks 1/8 inch by 1 inch

    1 garlic clove, minced

    1 tablespoon coconut oil

    Sea salt, pepper

    Fresh mint (optional)

1. Heat oil in a large skillet.
2. Put all ingredients into the skillet and sauté for 5–7 minutes or until fork tender but not too soft.
3. Season with salt and pepper.
4. Garnish with fresh mint if desired.

   Serves 4.

Dinner

SALMON CROQUETTES

My grandmother made these for me when I was little. My favorite thing was to hunt for the tiny, edible bones and crunch them. Now, I'm passing this recipe on to my children who love to do the same thing. We have contests to see who has the most bones, which are a great source of calcium.

1 can wild Alaskan salmon
½ cup quick-cooking oats
1 teaspoon Dijon mustard
1 farm-fresh egg
Pinch of dried dill
½ teaspoon sea salt
½ teaspoon ground pepper
1 tablespoon coconut oil or ghee

1. Put all the ingredients in a large bowl and use your hands to combine everything.
2. Form small patties with your hands.
3. Heat oil in a large skillet over medium heat.
4. Place croquettes in the skillet and brown on each side, about 3–4 minutes.

Tip: Serve with ketchup for the kids or try mixing a teaspoon of Sriracha with ketchup for a spicy kick.

Or mix a little honey with Dijon for a sweet and sour sauce.

Makes 6 croquettes.

FISH VERACRUZ

2 white fish filets, like Flounder
Juice of 1 lime
1 tablespoon olive oil
Sea salt
2 garlic cloves
1 small onion, diced
¼ cup white wine, fish stock or chicken stock
2 chopped tomatoes
2 bay leaves
1 teaspoon cumin
1 teaspoon oregano
½ cup pitted, halved olives
¼ cup capers

1. Squeeze juice on 1 lime on fish filets and sprinkle with salt.
2. Place in fridge for 20–30 minutes.
3. Heat oil in a medium skillet.
4. Saute onions.
5. Add garlic, chopped tomatoes, bay leaves, cumin, salt, oregano, olives and capers.
6. Add white wine or fish stock.
7. Add fish on top of sauce, cover and cook for about 10 minutes or until fish is flaky and done.

ASIAN CHICKEN AND FRIED RICE

1 cup of white or brown rice, cooked, cooled, fluffed with a fork
2–3 chicken breasts, cut into small cubes

2 tablespoons peanut or coconut oil

2 eggs, beaten

2 green onions, sliced

½ teaspoon ground ginger

2 teaspoon soy sauce

1 cup frozen peas and carrots (optional)

¼ cup chopped peanuts (optional)

Marinade

¼ cup sucanat or brown sugar

1 teaspoon ground ginger

¼ cup soy sauce

2 cloves crushed garlic

½ cup pineapple juice

Dash of crushed red pepper

1. Marinate chicken for 1–2 hours or overnight in the fridge with the marinade ingredients.
2. Heat 1 tablespoon oil in a large skillet or wok.
3. Cook chicken over medium high heat, stirring frequently.
4. Cook thoroughly and remove to a plate.
5. Add remaining tablespoon of oil to pan.
6. Add the cooled rice and green onions.
7. Stir-fry the rice by stirring around the pan swiftly.
8. Add ginger and soy sauce.
9. Move the rice to the sides of the pan, leaving the middle open.
10. Add the eggs and scramble, stir into the rice.
11. Add the peas and carrots and stir to cook (place a lid on top to steam the veggies).
13. Add the chicken back in to warm.

Serves 4-6.

ONE-POT SKINNY JAMBALAYA

1 pound organic chicken breast, cut into 1-inch cubes

½ pound uncooked wild shrimp, cleaned and tails removed

1 bunch of green onions, chopped (about 4–5 green onions);
reserve 2 tablespoons for garnish

1 red bell pepper, chopped

3 garlic cloves, minced

1 ½ cups tomato juice

14 ounce diced tomatoes (preferably jarred)

2 cups organic or homemade chicken broth

1 cup brown rice (rinsed)

1 teaspoon Cajun seasoning (or more if you like it spicy)

1 tablespoon olive oil

Hot sauce to taste

1. Heat olive oil in large skillet or paella pan over medium heat.
2. Add chicken and brown, about 3 minutes on each side.
3. Add scallions, peppers and garlic and cook for about 5 more minutes until veggies have softened.
4. Add in tomato juice, diced tomatoes, chicken broth, rice and Cajun seasoning.
5. Bring to a boil then lower heat and cover.
6. Cook 45 minutes or until rice is done, stirring occasionally.
7. Stir in shrimp at the very end and cook about 2 minutes until pink (shrimp doesn't take very long to cook) and then remove from heat.
8. Sprinkle with extra scallions and serve. You can add hot sauce to taste.

Serves 4-6.

Homemade Hamburger Helper—10-Minute Dinner

1. Saute diced **onion** and 1 minced **garlic** clove in a teaspoon of **olive oil**.
2. Brown 1 pound **ground beef**.
3. Add 2 cans **diced tomatoes**.
4. Sprinkle with **salt**, **pepper** and **Italian seasoning** blend.
5. Serve over elbow or bow-tie **pasta**.
6. Optional: add shredded cheddar cheese, parmesan cheese.

   Serves 3-4.

Broiled Salmon—10-Minute Dinner

1. Sprinkle **salt** and **pepper** over two **salmon** filets.
2. Variations for sauce: 2 tablespoons **honey**, 2 tablespoons **soy sauce**, squeeze of **lemon** juice OR 2 teaspoons **Dijon mustard**, 2 tablespoons **honey**, 2 tablespoons **soy sauce**.
3. Broil in oven on high for 10 min, 5 on each side. Serves 2.

Chicken Tacos—10-Minute Dinner

2–3 chicken breasts, sliced into tenders
1 red, yellow and orange bell pepper, sliced
1 red onion, sliced
½ teaspoon cumin
½ teaspoon garlic powder
½ teaspoon sea salt and pepper
1 tablespoon olive oil or ghee
8 corn tortillas

1. Season chicken breasts with salt, pepper, cumin and garlic powder.
2. Pan fry in a little olive oil or ghee, or grill them.
3. While the chicken is cooking, sauté the sliced bell pepper and onions.

4. Season the veggies with a little salt and pepper and any extra cumin and garlic.

5. Heat corn tortillas on a flat griddle till just brown.

6. Place chicken tenders in the tortilla and top with vegetables.

7. Top with your favorite topping:

   Toppings Bar

   Shredded cheese

   Diced avocado

   Fresh salsa

   Chopped cilantro

   Squeeze of lime juice

Serves 4.

Pesto Pasta—10-Minute Dinner

1–2 cups baby spinach

Handful walnuts or pine nuts

1 clove garlic

Juice of ½ lemon

¼ cup shredded pecorino romano (can also use parmesan)

Sea salt and pepper

¼ cup extra virgin olive oil

1. Blend all ingredients in a food processor, except the olive oil.

2. With machine still running, pour the olive oil through the top until combined.

3. Add pesto to warm cooked pasta.

Fish in Parchment

Flounder filet or other white, mild fish

Cut veggies of your choice: peppers, cherry tomatoes, zucchini, onions, mushrooms

Pinch of herbs like thyme, chives, oregano

Slice of lemon

Drizzle of olive oil

Sea salt and pepper

1. Place the fish and veggies on a piece of parchment about 12 inch by 15 inch.
2. Top with lemon slice, drizzle of oil, salt, pepper and herbs.
3. Tightly seal the packets.
4. Place on a baking sheet and bake at 450 degrees for 15–20 minutes.

CHICKEN PAD THAI

1 (16-ounce) package brown rice noodles

2 boneless, skinless chicken breasts, cut into thin strips

3 tablespoons coconut oil, divided

2 large eggs, beaten

1 tablespoon sucanat or brown sugar

3 tablespoons soy sauce or coconut aminos

1 tablespoon fish sauce

¼ teaspoon Sriracha sauce

1 tablespoon lime juice

1 tablespoon chopped garlic

½ cup chicken broth

1 carrot, grated

4 scallions, sliced thin

1 cup bean sprouts

¼ cup peanuts, coarsely chopped, for garnish

¼ cup fresh cilantro, roughly chopped, for garnish

1. Bring a large pot of water to a boil and turn off the heat.
2. Add the rice noodles and let them soften, about 7–10 minutes. Drain. In a small bowl, whisk together the sucanat, soy sauce, fish sauce, chile sauce, lime juice, garlic and broth. Set aside.
3. In a wok or a large skillet over high heat, add ½ tablespoon oil.

When hot, add the eggs and cook until they are firm. Remove them from the pan and let them cool a bit. Roughly chop them and set aside.

4. In the same wok or a large skillet over high heat, add 1 tablespoon of oil. Cook chicken until cooked through. Push chicken to the sides of the pan.

5. Add the remaining 1 tablespoon oil to the middle of the pan, add the carrots, scallions and bean sprouts.

6. Stir fry 1 minute.

7. Add the reserved eggs and sauce, stirring to coat everything completely.

8. Cook for another minute.

9. Serve over noodles and garnish with peanuts and cilantro.

Serves 4-6.

QUINOA, CARROT AND BUTTERNUT SQUASH STEW

Stew

2 tablespoons olive oil
1 cup chopped onion
3 garlic cloves, chopped
2 teaspoons paprika
1 teaspoon sea salt
½ teaspoon ground black pepper
½ teaspoon ground coriander
½ teaspoon ground cumin
½ teaspoon turmeric
½ teaspoon ground ginger
¼ teaspoon cayenne pepper (more if you like it very spicy)
1 cup water
1 (14.5-ounce) can diced tomatoes, drained
2 tablespoons fresh lemon juice

3 cups peeled butternut squash (from
1 ½-pound squash), 1-inch cubes

2 cups peeled carrots, ¾-inch cubes

Quinoa

1 cup quinoa, rinsed (rainbow quinoa makes for a very nice
presentation)

1 tablespoon butter or ghee

1 tablespoon olive oil

½ cup onion, finely chopped

2 garlic cloves, minced

½ teaspoon sea salt

½ teaspoon turmeric

2 cups water

¼ cup chopped fresh cilantro, divided

2 teaspoons chopped fresh mint, divided

For stew

1. Heat oil in large saucepan over medium heat.
2. Add onion; sauté until soft, stirring often, about 5 minutes.
3. Add garlic; stir 1 minute.
4. Mix in paprika and next 8 ingredients.
5. Add 1 cup water, tomatoes, and lemon juice. Bring to boil.
6. Add squash and carrots.
7. Cover and simmer over medium-low heat until vegetables are tender, stirring occasionally, about 20 minutes.
8. Season with salt and pepper.

Tip: This dish can be prepared one day ahead. Cover and chill.

For quinoa

1. Rinse quinoa; drain.
2. Melt butter with oil in large saucepan over medium heat.

3. Add onion and carrot.

4. Cover; cook until vegetables begin to brown, stirring often, about 10 minutes.

5. Add garlic, salt, and turmeric; sauté 1 minute.

6. Add quinoa; stir 1 minute.

7. Add 2 cups water. Bring to boil; reduce heat to medium-low.

8. Cover; simmer until liquid is absorbed and quinoa is tender, about 15 minutes.

9. Re-warm stew.

10. Stir in half of cilantro and half of mint.

11. Spoon quinoa onto platter, forming well in center. Spoon stew into well.

12. Sprinkle remaining herbs over.

Tip: This is a delicious and hearty vegan meal that can please all palates, vegan or not. It's also very pretty to serve with all the bright colors. Adapted from Bon Appetit.

Serves 6-8.

GRANDDAD'S MEATLOAF

    1 small onion, diced
    1 teaspoon olive oil
    2 pounds ground chuck, preferably grass-fed
    2 eggs
    $\frac{2}{3}$ cup ketchup
    1 ½ cups oats
    Dash each of thyme, garlic, cumin, rosemary
    1 teaspoon sea salt
    1 teaspoon ground pepper
    Tomato juice

1. Put olive oil in a medium small skillet and sauté the onions till tender.

2. Mix the cooled onions into all of the ingredients, except tomato juice.
3. Mix well with your hands.
4. Shape meatloaf mixture into 2 football-sized shapes.
5. Place both into a 13 x 9 baking pan.
6. Pour tomato juice over the meatloaf, just lining the bottom edges of the meatloaf.
7. Swirl ketchup on top to give it a glazed appearance.
8. Bake at 350 degrees for 1 hour.

Serves 4-5.

LIME MARINATED CHICKEN

Bunch of coarsely chopped fresh cilantro
1 crushed garlic clove
¾ cup olive oil
5 tablespoons fresh lime juice
2 ½ teaspoons ground cumin
1 ¼ teaspoons chili powder (ancho chili is best)
6 boneless chicken breasts or thighs

1. Combine the marinade ingredients together in a food processor or blender and pour over the chicken; place all in a plastic baggie.
2. Marinate for 3 to 4 hours in the fridge.
3. Remove chicken from the bag and season well with salt and pepper.
4. Grill on a preheated grill until the internal temperature reaches 165 degrees or about 7 minutes on each side for breasts and about 12 minutes per side for thighs.

Serves 6.

CHICKEN WITH LEMON BUTTER CAPER SAUCE

1 cup chicken stock
6 tablespoons lemon juice (juice of 2 lemons)
½ stick grass-fed butter
2 tablespoons capers
1 tablespoon arrowroot powder
½ cup cold water
Sea salt and pepper
4 chicken breasts
1 tablespoon olive oil or ghee

1. Slice chicken breasts into thinly-sliced pieces. Thinly sliced breasts will cook evenly and quicker.
2. Season chicken with salt and pepper.
3. Heat oil and cook chicken breasts over medium heat in a large skillet.
4. Melt ½ stick of butter over low heat in a saucepan.
5. Add 1 cup of chicken stock. Stir to combine and turn up the heat to medium-high.
6. Put arrowroot powder into a small bowl and add ½ cup of cold water, stir to combine.
7. Whisk in the arrowroot powder and bring to a low boil.
8. When the sauce is thickened (takes less than 1 minute), whisk in the lemon juice, 2 tbsp. at a time.
9. Stir in the capers. Season with salt and pepper to taste.
10. Pour the sauce over the plated chicken breasts.
11. Serve immediately.

Note: Could also be served over salmon or a white fish, like flounder.
Serves 4.

MOM'S SPAGHETTI SAUCE & MEATBALLS

Sauce

1 Vidalia or Texas Sweet onion, quartered

2 cloves garlic, minced

2 tablespoons olive oil

1 tablespoon Italian seasoning (see recipe section)

4 (14-ounce) cans tomato sauce

Meatballs

1 cup breadcrumbs

1 egg, beaten

1 pound ground chuck

½ teaspoon salt

½ teaspoon pepper

1 teaspoon Italian seasoning

1–2 tablespoons olive oil

1. Heat oil in a large soup pot or Dutch oven.
2. Add onion, minced garlic and Italian seasoning. Cook 1 minute until fragrant.
3. Add the tomato sauce and cook over low heat for 1 to 2 hours.

Meatball preparation

1. Mix all meatball ingredients (except olive oil) together and work the seasonings in with your hands.
2. Form into balls.
3. Heat olive oil in a large skillet.
4. Place meatballs into pan and fry, turning once to cook each side.
5. Place cooked meatballs into the pot with the spaghetti sauce.
6. Simmer for 1 hour.
7. Serve with brown rice pasta or whole-grain spaghetti noodles.

Serves 6.

Easy Chicken Enchiladas

    2–3 chicken breasts or utilize leftover chicken or turkey from a
        previous meal
    12 corn tortillas
    Pinches of salt, garlic powder and cumin
    3 pouches of Frontera Green Enchilada Sauce
    1 cup shredded cheddar cheese

1. Preheat oven to 350 degrees.
2. If your chicken is raw, place breasts in a pot of boiling water for 6–8 minutes and poach with lots of salt, garlic and cumin.
3. Remove and shred.
4. Place cooked, shredded chicken in a sauce pan with one pouch of Frontera enchilada sauce and warm.
5. Heat 4–5 tortillas at a time in a microwave for 30–40 seconds, wrapped in a paper towel.
6. Remove tortillas and, one-by-one, place a small spoonful of the chicken mixture into each tortilla.
7. Roll the tortillas and leave the seam side down in a 13 x 9 casserole dish.
8. Repeat the process until the chicken mixture is gone.
9. Pour the remaining two pouches of sauce on the enchiladas and sprinkle the top with shredded cheese.
10. Place into oven and bake for 15–20 minutes or until the cheese is melted.

    Serves 4.

Pork Tenderloin

    1–2 pork tenderloins, about 1 pound each
    2 tablespoons balsamic vinegar
    ½ teaspoon cumin

½ teaspoon ground ginger
½ teaspoon turmeric
½ teaspoon sea salt
½ teaspoon pepper
1 tablespoon coconut oil or olive oil

1. Rub marinade ingredients over pork tenderloins and place into a glass dish with a lid and marinate for 30 minutes to several hours.
2. Preheat oven to 400 degrees.
3. Heat 1 tablespoon oil in an oven-safe skillet.
4. Place tenderloins in a hot skillet to brown on each side.
5. Once browned, place the entire skillet into a hot oven and cook for 15–20 minutes.
6. Test with a meat thermometer and remove when pork reaches 145 degrees.
7. Let meat rest for 10 minutes for additional carry-over cooking.
8. Slice diagonally.

Serves 4, with leftovers.

Tip: Save leftovers for another meal, like my Honey Cashew Stir-fry or freeze one tenderloin for another time.

HONEY CASHEW PORK STIR-FRY OVER BROWN RICE

1 cup orange juice
½ cup honey
¼ cup soy sauce or Tamari
1 tablespoon coconut oil
¼ teaspoon ground ginger
3 carrots, sliced diagonally
1 bell pepper, sliced diagonally
6 boneless pork chops, OR utilize leftover pork tenderloin, cut into small pieces
⅔ cup cashews
Coconut oil for stir-frying

1. First, bring 2 ¼ cups of water, 1 ½ cups of brown rice and a heavy pinch of sea salt to a boil.
2. Reduce heat to low and cover and simmer 30–40 minutes or until tender and water is absorbed.
3. Combine orange juice, honey, soy sauce and ginger in a bowl. Set aside.
4. Heat the oil in a large skillet over medium-high heat.
5. Add the carrots and bell peppers and stir-fry until tender-crisp.
6. Remove the veggies and set aside.
7. Add more oil and stir-fry the pork until cooked through or reheat cut tenderloin leftovers.
8. Add the veggies back into the skillet, along with the sauce. Heat until it comes to a boil.
9. Add cashews at the very end to warm.
10. Serve over rice.

Serves 4.

BBQ CHICKEN PIZZA

½ cup prepared BBQ sauce
8-ounces chicken tenders or breasts, cut into bite-size pieces, cooked
¼ cup cilantro, chopped
2 slices red onion, cut into small pieces
1 cup mozzarella cheese, grated
½ cup smoked gouda (optional), grated
1 fresh pizza dough
EVOO

1. Roll out the pizza dough to your desired shape and thickness.
2. Brush the dough with a little EVOO.
3. Spread the BBQ sauce around the crust.
4. Spread all the toppings on top of the sauce.

5. Bake for 15–20 minutes at 400 degrees.

Serves 4.

COUNTRY-STYLE PORK RIBS

Dry Rub Ingredients

½ cup sucanat or brown sugar

1 teaspoon chili powder

1 teaspoon garlic powder

1 teaspoon paprika

1 teaspoon onion powder

1 teaspoon sea salt

1 teaspoon pepper

3–4 pounds pork ribs (country-style has more meat on it)

Prepared BBQ sauce

1. Rub the dry rub ingredients over the pork ribs.
2. Place on a baking sheet and cover with foil.
3. Bake for 1 hour at 350 degrees.
4. Pour off any liquid from the pan and brush the ribs with the BBQ sauce.
5. Cover with foil again and bake for another hour.
6. Take off foil for the last 20 minutes to brown.

Serves 4-6.

HOMEMADE CHICKEN NUGGETS

2–3 boneless, skinless chicken breasts, cut into 1-inch cubes

Choice of breading: 1 cup of breadcrumbs, almond meal or crushed bran flakes

Sea salt and pepper

1 egg, beaten

½ teaspoon Italian seasoning (optional)

Olive oil or ghee (if pan-frying)

1. Prepare your dredging stations: one large dish for the beaten egg and another for the breadcrumb mixture of salt, pepper and Italian seasoning. (A glass pie plate works well.)
2. Toss the chicken chunks into the egg mixture until they are coated on all sides. Season with salt and pepper.
3. Using one hand, place a few chicken pieces in the dry, breadcrumb mix and toss to coat.
4. Place the coated chicken on a clean plate while you bread the rest of the chicken.
5. Heat oil in a large skillet and pan fry the nuggets until they are golden brown.

Serves 4.

Tip: Alternatively, you can bake in the oven for 20 minutes on 350 degrees. Place chicken pieces on a baking sheet. Turning once.

HOMEMADE FISH STICKS

2–3 filets of flounder or cod, cut into 4-inch strips
Choice of breading: 1 cup of breadcrumbs, almond meal or
    crushed bran flakes
Sea salt and pepper
1 egg, beaten
½ teaspoon garlic powder
Olive oil or ghee (if pan-frying)

1. Prepare your dredging stations: one large dish for the beaten egg and another for the breadcrumb mixture of salt, pepper and garlic powder. (A glass pie plate works well.)
2. Gently place the fish strips into the egg mixture until they are coated on all sides. Season with salt and pepper.
3. Using one hand, place a few pieces in the dry, breadcrumb mix and toss to coat. Place the coated fish on a clean plate while you

bread the rest of the fish.

4. Heat oil in a large skillet and pan fry until they are golden brown.

Serves 4.

Tip: Alternatively, you can bake in the oven for 20 minutes on 350 degrees. Place fish pieces on a baking sheet. Turning once with a spatula. Remove when golden brown.

CHICKEN WINGS TWO WAYS
2 dozen chicken wings
Salt, pepper, paprika, ground ginger, olive oil

HONEY BBQ
½ cup prepared BBQ sauce (see recipe section)
1 teaspoon raw honey

Hot Buffalo Wings—Frank's RedHot Sauce

1. Place chicken wings in a large bowl.
2. Sprinkle with salt, pepper, paprika, ginger and a dash of olive oil.
3. Toss to coat.
4. Place onto a baking sheet.
5. Put into a 400-degree oven for 50–55 minutes, turning once.
6. When cooked, remove and place half of the wings in one large bowl and half in another bowl.
7. Pour BBQ and honey over the wings in one bowl and the hot sauce in another bowl. Toss to coat the wings.

Serves 3-4.

BAKED DRUMSTICKS

1. Sprinkle salt, pepper, garlic powder and paprika over 8–10 drumsticks.
2. Place on a baking sheet.
3. Drizzle with a small amount of olive oil or avocado oil.
4. Bake for 375 degrees for 50–60 minutes, depending on the size of your drumsticks; turn over after 30 minutes. Serves 4.

Tip: You can eat them as is when they're done or douse with hot sauce or Honey BBQ sauce for the kids.

GROUND BEEF THREE WAYS

Easy Nachos

1. Brown 1 pound ground **beef**, drain grease.
2. Stir in 1 (14-ounce) can diced **tomatoes** and add seasonings of your choice (Italian, Mexican)
3. Add one can drained and rinsed **black beans**.
4. Cook off the liquid from the tomatoes.
5. Layer the beef mixture on top of the tortilla chips for nachos or inside corn tortillas for tacos.
6. Top with organic **shredded cheese**, **fresh salsa** and **diced avocado. Serves 4.**

Stuffed Peppers

1. Brown 1 pound ground **beef** and ½ diced **onion**. Drain grease.
2. Add **salt, pepper** and **garlic powder**.
3. Stir in 4 ounces of **tomato sauce** and 1 cup cooked **rice**.
4. Spoon mixture into 4 **sweet bell peppers** with the tops and ribs removed.
5. Place in a baking pan and bake at 350 degrees for 25–30 minutes. **Serves 4.**

Grass-fed Burgers

1. Grate ½ medium **onion** into fine mince.
2. Mix 1 pound grass-fed **beef** with finely grated onion, ½ teaspoon each of **garlic powder**, sea **salt**, **pepper** and **onion powder**.
3. Form into 4 patties.
4. Grill 3–4 minutes on each side. **Serves 4.**

Tip: Grass-fed beef is leaner than grain-fed beef. The grated onion helps to add moisture.

CHICKEN BREAST THREE WAYS

Baked Chicken Parmesan

1. Coat 3–4 **chicken breasts** in 1 beaten **egg**.
2. Dredge through a mixture of **breadcrumbs** seasoned with dried oregano, basil, thyme, salt and pepper.
3. Place breaded breasts on a baking sheet and put into oven at 350 degrees for 20–25 minutes.
4. When chicken is done, spoon 1 tablespoon **marinara sauce** on each breast and sprinkle with **shredded mozzarella cheese**.
5. Return to oven for 5 minutes. Finish with freshly grated parmesan cheese. **Serves 4.**

Chicken and Vegetable Stir-fry

1. Cut **chicken** into bite-sized pieces.
2. Place into a large hot skillet with **oil** or ghee and sauté.
3. Toss in roughly **chopped broccoli**, **bell peppers**, **carrots**, **onions**, **mushrooms** (whatever veggies you like) and sauté.
4. Add in your favorite **seasonings** (Italian, Indian, Asian or Greek).
5. Serve over rice or quinoa. **Serves 4.**

Chicken on a Stick

1. Cut **chicken** into cubes and marinate in your favorite **seasonings** with a little bit of **olive oil** and **lemon** or **lime juice**.
2. Marinate for at least 30 minutes in the fridge.
3. Place chicken on a skewer that has been soaked in water for 10 minutes.
4. Grill for 4–5 min on each side.
5. Serve with honey Dijon or peanut satay sauce.

WILD SALMON THREE WAYS

Tip: Choose wild Alaskan salmon instead of farmed or Atlantic.

Honey Dijon Salmon

1. Marinate 4 **salmon** filets in 1 tablespoon **Dijon mustard**, 1 tablespoon **honey** and 2 tablespoons **soy sauce.**
2. Drizzle with **olive oil.**
3. Place in the fridge for 10–15 minutes.
4. Grill salmon for 4–5 min, starting with the skin side down.
5. Flip and sear the top for 1–2 minutes.
6. Sprinkle with salt and pepper. **Serves 4.**

Salmon in Parchment

1. Place **salmon** filet on top of a large square of parchment paper.
2. Season with **salt, pepper, garlic powder** and fresh **dill** and place a thin slice of **lemon** on top.
3. Top with sliced **zucchini** or **artichoke hearts** and **cherry tomatoes**.
4. Squeeze juice of ½ lemon over the top.
5. Fold over the parchment and seal edges.
6. Place packets on a baking sheet in a 400-degree oven for 15 minutes. **Serves 1.**

Pan-fried Salmon

1. Place **salmon** filet in a hot cast iron skillet with 1 tablespoon melted **ghee**.
2. Season with **salt, pepper, garlic powder** and fresh or dried **dill**.
3. Pan-fry for 4–5 minutes.
4. Flip and sear top for 1–2 minutes. **Serves 1.**

PASTA THREE WAYS

Pasta with Tuna & Peas

1. Cook 1 pound **corkscrew pasta** noodles and drain, reserving ½ cup of pasta water.
2. Add 1 can of **tuna**, broken up; ¾ cup frozen, thawed **peas**; and 1 tablespoon **olive oil** to hot pasta.
3. Pour ½ cup pasta water and 1 tablespoon **ghee** over the top to form a sauce.
4. Season with **salt, pepper, garlic powder** and **thyme**.
5. Sprinkle with grated **parmesan** or **pecorino romano cheese**. **Serves 3-4.**

Quick Shrimp with Linguine

1. In a large skillet, heat 2 tablespoons butter or **ghee** over medium heat.
2. Add 1 pound **wild shrimp** (peeled) to 2–3 cloves minced **garlic** and sauté until pink.
3. Squeeze juice of 1 **lemon** over the shrimp.
4. Add chopped fresh **parsley**, **salt** and **pepper**.
5. Serve over warm **linguine**. **Serves 4.**

Greek Orzo Pasta Salad

1. Cook ¾ cup **orzo** pasta.
2. Combine 1 tablespoon **olive oil**, 1 tablespoon **red wine vinegar**, sea **salt**, and **pepper** in a large bowl, stirring with a whisk.
3. Add orzo, 1 diced and seeded **tomato**, ½ cup chopped **bell pepper**, ½ diced **red onion**.
4. Sprinkle with chopped, fresh **parsley**, and 4 **Castelvetrano olives**, sliced.
5. Stir to combine.
6. Top with crumbled **feta cheese**. **Serves 4.**

SLOW-COOKER THREE WAYS

Chicken Taco Soup

1. Place 4 boneless **chicken thighs** into a slow cooker.
2. Mix together a 4-ounce can of diced **green chiles**, 2 cloves minced **garlic**, 1 diced **onion** and 2 cans **diced tomatoes**.
3. Stir in 1 cup **chicken broth**, 1 teaspoon **cumin**, **salt** and **pepper**.
4. Cook on high for 3 hours.
5. Shred chicken with a fork when tender.
6. Add more broth if needed.
7. Serve in soup bowls with **cilantro**, **lime juice** and **shredded cheese**. **Serves 4-6.**

Pork Shoulder Carnitas

1. Place a 2–3 pound **shoulder roast** in a slow cooker that has been rubbed liberally with **cumin**, **garlic powder**, **chili powder**, **onion powder**, **salt**, **pepper** and **oregano**.
2. Squeeze juice of 1 **lime** over the top and pour 1 cup of **water** around the bottom of the roast.
3. Cook on low for 6–8 hours.

4. Shred with a fork when done.

5. Use for tacos, nachos or serve over rice. **Serves 4-6.**

Pot Roast

1. Place a 3–4 pound **chuck roast** into a slow cooker that has been seasoned with **salt, pepper, garlic powder, onion powder** and **thyme** (place on top of 2 sliced **onions** to form a bed).

2. Pour 1–2 cups **beef broth** (or chicken broth in a pinch) and a splash of **balsamic vinegar**.

3. Place 4–5 peeled and roughly chopped **carrots** and 4–5 peeled **potatoes**, cut into large chunks, around the beef.

4. Cook on low for 8 hours.

5. Season with more salt and pepper to taste when done. **Serves 4-6.**

Snacks & Sweet Treats

STOVE-TOP POPCORN

¼ cup organic popcorn kernels
1 tablespoon coconut oil
Sea Salt

1. In a saucepan, melt the oil over medium heat.

2. Pour in the popcorn and cover immediately.

3. Shake the pan over the heat to coat the kernels.

4. Keep shaking every 15–20 seconds, or until the popping has stopped.

5. After the popcorn has popped, pour into a large bowl.
   Serves 4.

FLAVORED POPCORN

Sweet: Sprinkle cinnamon, sugar and sea salt on top. Toss to coat.

Garlic: Garlic powder, onion powder and sea salt

Curry: Curry powder and sea salt

Spicy: Chili powder, cumin, garlic powder and red chili flakes

MICROWAVE POPCORN

1. Place ¼ cup organic popcorn kernels in a brown paper bag.
2. Fold over the bag to close tightly.
3. Microwave on high for about 2 minutes.
4. Stand near the microwave. When you hear the popping stop, immediately stop the microwave or it will burn.
5. Dump into a large bowl.

Serves 4.

Tip: You can add melted butter or ghee and sea salt for a movie theater-style taste.

Tip: Don't have a brown paper bag? Place ¼ cup popcorn in a glass Pyrex bowl and place a microwave-safe ceramic plate on top. Microwave for about 2 to 2 ½ minutes. Stop when the popping has stopped. The bowl will be hot. Use oven mitts to remove.

CHERRY CHOCOLATE PROTEIN BITES

Prep time: 5 minutes, Prep notes: 15 minutes to roll about 30–40 balls

    2 cups quick cooking rolled oats
    dash Celtic sea salt
    ½ cup dried tart cherries
    1 cup pitted Medjool dates
    1 tablespoon chia seeds
    4 tablespoons natural peanut butter (sun butter or any nut
        butter will do)

1 teaspoon vanilla extract

1 teaspoon cinnamon

¼ cup mini chocolate chips (preferably semi-sweet, milk-free)

1. Put oats and salt in a food processor.
2. Process until finely ground.
3. Add remaining ingredients, except for chocolate chips, and process until fully combined.
4. Add ½ teaspoon water to bring ingredients together.
5. Fold in chocolate chips.
6. Add a few drops of water if needed to form balls.
7. Form into balls or press into a square pan and cut into squares.

Tip: Makes 40–50 balls depending on how big you make each one. Keep in the fridge in an airtight container. If you want a more distinct cherry taste, chop the cherries instead of processing in the food processor. You'll have bigger chunks in each ball.

* Don't be tempted to leave out the amazing little chia seeds. These suckers are packed with fiber, protein, omega-3's and tons of nutrients! You can put them in smoothies, oatmeal, sauces, water, pudding and more!

PEANUT BUTTER PROTEIN BALLS

1 cup quick cooking rolled oats

Dash Celtic sea salt

½ cup organic raisins

½ cup pitted Medjool dates

2 tablespoons natural peanut butter (okay to substitute with sun butter to make it nut-free)

1 teaspoon vanilla extract

½ teaspoon cinnamon

1. Put oats and salt in a food processor.
2. Process until finely ground.
3. Add remaining ingredients and process until fully combined.
4. Add a few drops of water, if needed for stickiness.
5. Form into balls or press into a square pan and cut into squares.

Tip: Makes 20–30 balls depending on how big you make them.

HOMEMADE GRANOLA BARS

½ cup favorite nut butter (cashew and almond are best, but
   peanut butter will do)
⅓ cup raw, local honey
¼ cup virgin, unrefined coconut oil
1 cup quick cooking oats
1 ½ cups raw nuts and seeds
Dash of cinnamon
Optional: ¼ cup of raisins, dried cherries or chocolate chips

1. Melt the nut butter, honey and oil over VERY low heat so as not to destroy the live enzymes in the honey. Stir to combine. This just takes 1–2 minutes.
2. Pour this warm mixture over 1 cup of quick cooking oats, 1 ½ cups nuts and seeds.*
3. Add mix-ins. This could be organic raisins, dried cherries, dried fruit or chocolate chips (up to ¼ cup). I like to add a generous sprinkle of cinnamon too!
4. Stir to combine.
5. Pour into a square brownie pan lined with parchment paper, press down and chill for 30 min to 1 hr.
6. Store in an air-tight container in the fridge.

  * I use a mixture of the following raw, unsalted and sprouted nuts and seeds: Raw almonds, Brazil nuts, raw pumpkin and sunflower

seeds, chia seeds, ground flax seeds, cashews, walnuts. All are chopped coarsely, though I leave the pumpkin and sunflower seeds whole.

Tip: For a grain-free version, use more nuts and seeds and skip the oats.

Tip: For a nut-free version, use lots of pumpkin, chia, flax and sunflower seeds as well as more oats.

Makes 12 bars.

Molten Lava Chocolate Cake

Note: 5 minutes to prep, 10 min to cook.

 4 tablespoons unsalted ghee or grass-fed butter, plus more for greasing the ramekins

 1 tablespoon gluten-free flour, plus more for dusting the ramekins (I like Bob's Red Mill or just brown rice flour). You can use unbleached flour as well.

 ⅓ cup bittersweet chocolate chips (I like Enjoy Life's dairy-free chips)

 1 large egg, plus 1 large egg yolk

 2 tablespoons sucanat, coconut palm sugar or pure cane sugar

1. Preheat oven to 450 degrees.
2. Prepare the ramekins: butter (or you can use coconut oil) two 6-ounce ramekins and dust with GF or regular flour.
3. Place the butter and chocolate chips in a glass bowl and microwave on high in 20-second intervals, stirring after each, until melted. Alternately, you can place the butter and chocolate chips in a glass bowl over a pan of simmering water on low heat. Stir till melted.
4. Using an electric mixer, beat the egg, egg yolk and sucanat in a medium bowl until thick, about 1 minute.
5. Add the melted chocolate and flour and beat until smooth.

6. Divide the batter between the two prepared ramekins. Bake until edges are set and center is still jiggly, about 8–10 minutes.

7. Let stand for 15 seconds and then run a knife around the edges. Invert onto a small plate.

8. Serve with small berries or make a sauce with crushed berries and drizzle on top. You can prepare these ahead of time by placing the batter in the ramekins in the fridge for 1 day. Bring to room temp before baking.

Serves 2.

HOMEMADE MARSHMALLOWS

Marshmallows from the store are highly processed and full of the Nasty 9 ingredients. I love making homemade marshmallows for my kids. They also make great gifts around the holidays.

¼ cup Great Lakes gelatin (found on Amazon.com)
1 cup ice cold water, divided
1 ½ cups granulated, pure cane sugar
½ cup real maple syrup
Pinch sea salt
1 teaspoon vanilla extract
¼ cup powdered sugar
¼ cup arrowroot powder
Nonstick spray (without butane as a propellant)

1. Place the gelatin into the bowl of a stand mixer along with ½ cup of the water. Use the whisk attachment. In a small saucepan combine the remaining ½ cup water, granulated sugar, maple syrup and salt.

2. Place over medium-high heat, cover and allow to cook for 3–4 minutes.

3. Uncover, clip a candy thermometer onto the side of the pan

and continue to cook until the mixture reaches 240 degrees, approximately 10 minutes. Immediately remove from the heat.

4. Turn the mixer on low speed and, while running, slowly pour the syrup down the side of the bowl into the gelatin mixture. Once you have added all of the syrup, increase the speed to high.

5. Continue to whip until the mixture becomes very thick, approximately 10–12 minutes.

6. Add the vanilla during the last minute of whipping.

7. While the mixture is whipping prepare the pan as follows:

   - Combine the powdered sugar and arrowroot powder in a small bowl. Lightly spray a 13 by 9-inch metal baking pan with nonstick cooking spray. Add the sugar and arrowroot mixture and move around to completely coat the bottom and sides of the pan. Reserve the remaining sugar mixture to the bowl for later use.

   - When ready, pour the marshmallow mixture into the prepared pan using a lightly oiled spatula for spreading evenly into the pan. Allow the marshmallows to sit uncovered for at least 4 hours to cure.

   - Turn the marshmallows out onto a large cutting board (dusted with the remaining sugar/starch mixture) and cut into 1-inch squares using a pizza wheel dusted with the powdered sugar mixture. Once cut, lightly dust all sides of each marshmallow with the remaining mixture, using additional if necessary. Store in an airtight container for up to 3 weeks. Makes 3-4 dozen.

Tip: Want peppermint flavored marshmallows? Try adding 1–2 drops of food-grade peppermint oil to the last stages of whipping. These are great for hot cocoa!

Summer Berry Popsicles

    1 handful of fresh spinach
    1 cup of strawberries, blueberries and/or raspberries
    1 cup of almond or coconut milk

1. Blend all of the ingredients in a high-powered blender.
2. Pour into popsicle molds and freeze. Makes 4-6 popsicles.

Healthy Snack Ideas

- Almonds, walnuts or cashews (a small palm-ful is usually a serving)
- Sunflower seeds and raisins
- Celery and nut butter (or sun butter), 1–2 tablespoons
- Rice chips, veggies with hummus
- Organic tortilla chips and salsa or guacamole (for those that just have to have chips). Plaintain chips are yummy too!
- Veggie sticks (celery, carrots, cucumber) with hummus or guacamole
- Kale chips (make your own)
- Zucchini oven chips (make your own)
- Sweet potato chips or fries (make your own)
- Apple slices with nut butter or sun butter
- Pumpkin seeds and dried cranberries
- Greek yogurt with granola (IF you tolerate dairy. Read labels to avoid high-fructose corn syrup, artificial colors and sweeteners)
- Green smoothie with flax or chia seeds
- Fresh fruit or fruit salad
- Make your own trail mix with raw nuts seeds and dried fruit
- Pumpkin smoothie (pumpkin puree, almond milk, chia seeds, honey, cinnamon, almonds and ½ banana)
- Dinner leftovers
- Salad with a variety of vegetables and olive oil-based dressing

- For an easy on-the-go snack, check out Lara Bars (get the ones without added sugar).
- Mixed berries (or mixed berry smoothie with flax seeds or chia seeds)

Drinks

FLAVORED WATER

Not a fan of plain water? Try upgrading your water by adding one of the following:

Sliced cucumber

Sliced oranges

Lemon or lime slices

Peppermint essential oil

Berries

Mint leaves

Sprig of fresh rosemary

HOT CHOCOLATE

2 cups of almond or coconut milk

3 tablespoons real maple syrup

2 tablespoons raw cacao (Navitas brand is good)

Splash of vanilla extract

Dash of cinnamon

1. Slowly warm the milk in a saucepan.
2. Whisk in the rest of the ingredients.
3. Serve with homemade marshmallows. Serves 4.

PUMKPIN ROOIBOS TEA

2–3 Yogi Chai Rooibos tea bags, steeped in 12–16 ounces of very hot water for 5 minutes.

2 tablespoons fresh, pure pumpkin

½ teaspoon pumpkin pie spice

Heavy dashes of cinnamon

Pinch sea salt

1 teaspoon vanilla extract

10 drops liquid Stevia, or to taste (raw honey is okay to use)

½ cup almond or coconut milk

1. Steep the tea.
2. Blend all ingredients in a blender.
3. Serve immediately while warm and frothy.

Serves 2.

CUCUMBER JUICE

Run the following items through your juicer:

1 cucumber

1–2 stalks of organic celery

1 apple

½ lemon

1 carrot

Serves 2.

CHOCOLATE SMOOTHIE SENSATION

1 banana

1 handful baby spinach (preferably organic)

1 teaspoon ground flax seeds

1 teaspoon chia seeds

1 teaspoon maca powder (great for enhancing libido)

1 tablespoon raw cacao

1 cup coconut or almond milk

1 tablespoon high-quality protein powder (True Whey brand is good)

½ cup organic frozen fruit of your choice

1. Blend spinach, seeds and milk.
2. Blend in remaining ingredients.

Tip: You can add ice if you like it extra cold!

Serves 1.

Basics

HOMEMADE CHICKEN STOCK (BONE BROTH)

Save your beef bones, oxtail, turkey carcass or chicken bones when you consume them. Toss any leftover bones in the freezer if you don't have time to make broth right away. When you're ready to make broth, there are three ways to cook it. These methods make a plain, unsalted stock that you can therefore use in any recipe.

METHOD 1: SLOW-COOKER

1. Put **bones** in a large slow-cooker and let sit for 30 minutes with 1–2 tablespoons **raw apple cider vinegar** (like Bragg's brand). This helps draw the minerals out of the bones.
2. Throw in an **onion**, a couple **celery** ribs, 2 **carrots**.
3. Cover bones with water (veggies are optional).
4. You could also save your extra veggie scraps and toss those in a freezer for later broth making.
5. Set the slow-cooker on low and go through 2 cycles for 8–10 hours each. Total cooking time will be about 20–24 hours, depending on your settings.
6. The bones are "done" when they crumble in between your fingers.

Tip: In the winter time, I will make broth all week long using the same bones. I will remove the finished stock, add more water to the bones and continue the process for another 24 hours. I use the broth to make soups and any recipe calling for chicken or beef stock.

Method 2: Stove-Top

1. Put **bones** in a large stock pot and let sit for 30 minutes with 1–2 tablespoons **raw apple cider vinegar.**
2. Throw in an **onion**, a couple **celery** ribs and 2 **carrots**.
3. Cover bones with water (veggies are optional).
4. Let it come to a slow boil.
5. Turn the heat down to low and simmer for a minimum of 8–24 hours for chicken, 10–24 hours for beef or 4–24 hours for fish stock. This is not my preferred method due to the excessive amount of time the stove is left on.

Method 3: Instant Pot

Tip: Use an electric pressure cooker—my favorite method!

1. Place **bones** into pressure cooker pot.
2. Fill with filtered water to the maximum line.
3. Add 1 tablespoon **raw apple cider vinegar**. Let sit for 30 minutes.
4. Veggies are optional.
5. Place lid on top and set timer for 90 minutes.
6. Contents will come to up to pressure and then the timer will start.
7. When cooking is done, allow the pressure cooker to release steam naturally, about 10 minutes.

Tip: For all three cooking methods, remove the stock by ladling into glass mason jars. I use a mesh strainer to keep out the smaller bones and cartilage. Set the jars on the counter to cool down before placing in the fridge. I don't skim the fat until the stock has completely gelled or cooled in the fridge. This protective layer of fat also allows for your stock to stay fresh in the fridge longer. It is nature's own natural preservative!

Tip: Store for 5–7 days in the fridge. Use for soups and drinking as well as braising liquid for making greens. Store for up to 6 months in the freezer in BPA-free plastic canning jars or glass mason jars with 2 inches of headspace to allow for expansion.

Fun Note: Chicken feet make your stock very nutritious and gelatinous! Don't be scared to get a few from your farmer.

ITALIAN SEASONING
   3 tablespoons dried basil
   3 tablespoons dried oregano
   3 tablespoons dried parsley
   1 tablespoon garlic powder
   1 teaspoon onion powder
   1 teaspoon dried thyme
   1 teaspoon dried rosemary
   1 teaspoon dried marjoram
   1 teaspoon red pepper flakes
   ¼ teaspoon black pepper

1. Mix all ingredients in a spice grinder OR put in a small bowl and crush with the back of a spoon.
2. Store in an airtight jar for up to 6 months.

CHILI POWDER
   2 teaspoons paprika
   4 teaspoons cumin
   2 teaspoons cayenne
   2 teaspoons oregano
   4 teaspoons garlic powder

1. Mix together.
2. Store in a small glass jar with your spices.

HOMEMADE TACO SEASONING

2 tablespoons chili powder
5 teaspoons paprika
4 teaspoons ground cumin
3 teaspoons onion powder
2 ½ teaspoons garlic powder
2 teaspoons sea salt
⅛ teaspoon cayenne pepper

1. Combine seasonings into an airtight container. This will keep for about a year . . . but I don't think it will be around that long.
2. When making taco meat: cook 1 pound of meat until no longer brown. Add ¾ cup water and 2 ½ tablespoons of seasoning. Bring to a quick boil, reduce heat and simmer until liquid is absorbed (about 10 minutes).

QUICK BBQ SAUCE

1 cup ketchup (read label for HFCS)
¼ cup apple cider vinegar
½ cup molasses or maple syrup
½ teaspoon salt
1 teaspoon worcestershire sauce
¼ teaspoon garlic powder
¼ teaspoon onion powder
¼ teaspoon black pepper

1. Whisk over medium-high heat in a saucepan.
2. Boil for 1 minute.
3. Simmer for 20 minutes.

You did it!

I hope this book inspires and empowers you to create change in your life – however small the steps may be. You now have the tools and knowledge to make informed decisions about what your family will consume and what you will put on your body. I want to hear from you. Did making these changes help you feel better, lose weight, sleep more soundly or lower your cholesterol? Share it with your friends and family and help them discover these tools as well. Together we can create massive change in the food world!

Chapter 14: Resources for Healthy Living

Find healthy food near you

Localharvest.org. Search for local farmers' markets, CSAs and farms near you.

Eatwild.com. Find grass-fed, pastured meats as well as eggs and dairy near you.

PickYourOwn.org. Find a pick-your-own farm near you.

Farmersmarketcoalition.org. Connects consumers with farmers and farm markets.

Healthy food delivery

Vitacost.com. Find supplements, whole foods and personal care products at a discount.

Amazon.com. Their Subscribe and Save program can save you money.

ThriveMarket.com. Find healthy food at deep discounts.

VitalChoice.com. Find sustainable seafood.

Eating well on the road

Eatwellguide.org. Helps you find over 25,000 local, healthy establishments.

GMO resources

GMOinside.org. Information and tools to learn more about GMOs.

JustLabelIt.org. Grass-roots advocates helping to get GMOs labeled.

Nongmoproject.org. Non-profit organization offering third-party verification and labeling of non-GMO foods and products.

Food advocacy groups and watchdogs

OrganicConsumers.org. Organic Consumers Association. Non-profit campaigning for health, food safety and corporate accountability.

EWG.org. Environmental Working Group. Non-profit organization providing thorough research and information on pesticides, toxins in our environment and food, and numerous databases for safer products.

Apps for healthy living

BETTER SLEEP

Twilight (Android, iOS). Dims your screen to reduce blue light and eyestrain if you have to use the phone late at night!

Sleep Cycle (Android and iOS). An intelligent alarm clock that analyzes your sleep and wakes you in the lightest sleep phase.

SleepBot (Android and iOS). Alarm plus, record your movements and sounds during the night to wake up better each morning during light sleep.

FOOD TRACKING

MyFitnessPal (Android, iOS and Windows Phone). Track your diet and exercise.

FatSecret (Android, iOS and Windows Phone). Nutritional information for the food you eat and tracks your meals, exercise and weight.

Sparkpeople (Android, iOS). Fitness tracking and calorie counting tools, exercise demos, and more.

Meal Logger (Android). Tracks your food and exercise.

Lose It (Android). Use for exercise and food tracking; food preferences.

Cooking and shopping

GroceryIQ (Android, iOS). This app will let you share with everyone in your family for easy meal planning.

Out of Milk (Android). Shopping list, pantry list and to-do list, plus sharing capabilities.

Food Planner (Android). Lets you add planned meals, recipes, groceries and more.

Eating out

Find Me GF (Android). Find a Gluten-free restaurant or menu items near you.

HealthyOut (Android, iOS). A generic location app for all kinds of special diet requirements.

PaleoGoGo (Android, iOS). A Paleo-specific app that helps you find healthy food at US chain restaurants.

Recipe apps

The Wellness Mama (Android, iOS). Wellness information, recipes, remedies.

Nom Nom Paleo (iPad only). Paleo recipes, photos and cooking instructions.

STRESS MANAGEMENT
Headspace (Android). Meditation and mindfulness techniques in just 10 minutes a day.

Apps to help with workouts

RunKeeper (Android, iOS). Tracks your runs.

CROSSFIT SPECIFIC APPS:
Beyond the Whiteboard (Android, iOS)

WOD Tracker (Android only)

myWOD (Android, iOS).

Sworkit (Android, iOS). Lets you choose your body part and automatically creates bodyweight circuit training workouts.

Food information

Fooducate (Android). Scan a food item's barcode to get a rating and a healthier suggestion.

EWG Food Scores (Android, iOS). Rates more than 80,000 foods on a scale.

Dirty Dozen (Android, iOS). EWG Guide to the Dirty Dozen and Clean 15—a must for your smartphone!

Seafood Watch (Android, iOS). Search for safe seafood to eat; sushi guide from the Monterey Bay Aquarium.

Bibliography

1. Gaetano Di Chiara, Valentina Bassareo. "Reward System and Addiction: What Dopamine Does and Doesn't Do." *Science Direct.* N.p., Apr. 2007. Web. 03 Mar. 2015.

2. "From Passive Overeating to 'Food Addiction': A Spectrum of Compulsion and Severity." *From Passive Overeating to "Food Addiction": A Spectrum of Compulsion and Severity.* N.p., 2013. Web. 24 Feb. 2015.

3. "Result Filters." *National Center for Biotechnology Information.* U.S. National Library of Medicine, 2013. Web. 24 Feb. 2015.

4. "Ogden CL, Carroll MD, Kit BK, Flegal KM. Prevalence of Obesity and Trends in Body Mass Index among US Children and Adolescents," 1999–2010. JAMA. 2012:307:483–90. Web.

5. "Flegal KM, Carroll MD, Kit BK, Ogden CL. Prevalence of Obesity and Trends in the Distribution of Body Mass Index among US Adults," 1999–2010. JAMA. 2012:307:491–7. Web.

6. "5 Surprising Factors Why You May Be Gaining Weight." Mercola.com. Web. 24 Feb. 2015.

7. Web. Murphy SL, Xu JQ, Kochanek KD. Deaths: Final data for 2010. Natl Vital Stat Rep. 2013:61(4).

8. *Centers for Disease Control and Prevention.* Centers for Disease Control and Prevention, 02 June 2009. Web. 24 Feb. 2015. http://www.cdc.gov/nchs/data/nvsr/nvsr61/nvsr61_04.pdf[PDF-3M].

9. "GMO Facts." *The NonGMO Project RSS.* Web. 11 Feb. 2015. http://www.nongmoproject.org/learn-more/.

10. "Mazaya Theme." *Mortality in Sheep Flocks after Grazing on Bt Cotton Fields Warangal District, Andhra Pradesh.* Web. 24 Feb. 2015. http://gmwatch.org/latest-listing/1-news-items/6416-mortality-in-sheep-flocks-after-grazing-on-bt-cotton-fields-warangal-district-andhra-pradesh-2942006.

11. "Institute for Responsible Technology." Web. 24 Feb. 2015. http://www.responsibletechnology.org/health-risks#endref1.

12. "Genetically Modified Foods." *Position Paper:: The American Academy of Environmental Medicine (AAEM).* N.p., n.d. Web. 24 Feb. 2015. http://www.aaemonline.org/gmopost.html.

13. Hye-Yung Yum, Soo-Young Lee, Kyung-Eun Lee, Myung-Hyun Sohn,

Kyu-Earn Kim, "Genetically Modified and Wild Soybeans: An Immuno-logic Comparison," *Allergy and Asthma Proceedings 26, No. 3* (May–June 2005): 210–216(7). (2005): n. pag.

14. M. Green, et al., "Public health implications of the microbial pesticide Bacillus thuringiensis: An epidemiological study, Oregon, 1985–86," *Amer. J. Public Health 80,* no. 7(1990): 848–852; and M.A. Noble, P.D. Riben, and G. J. Cook, Microbiological and epidemiological surveillance program to monitor the health effects of Foray 48B BTK spray (Vancouver, B.C.: Ministry of Forests, Province of British Columbia, Sep. 30, 1992).

15. Vazquez et al, "Intragastric and intraperitoneal administration of Cry1Ac protoxin from Bacillus thuringiensis induces systemic and mucosal antibody responses in mice," 1897–1912; Vazquez et al, "Characterization of the mucosal and systemic immune response induced by Cry1Ac protein from Bacillus thuringiensis HD 73 in mice," *Brazilian Journal of Medical and Biological Research* 33 (2000): 147–155; and Vazquez et al, "Bacillus thuringiensis Cry1Ac protoxin is a potent systemic and mucosal adjuvant," *Scandanavian Journal of Immunology* 49 (1999): 578–584. See also Vazquez-Padron et al., 147 (2000b).

16. Fares, Nagui H., and Adel K. El-Sayed. "Fine Structural Changes in the Ileum of Mice Fed on Endotoxin-Treated Potatoes and Transgenic Potatoes." *Natural Toxins* 6.6 (1998): 219–33.

17. "Scientists Need to Rethink Their Beliefs about GMOs." *Des Moines Register.* N.p., n.d. Web. 24 Feb. 2015. http://www.desmoinesregister.com/story/opinion/columnists/2014/12/15/scientists-need-rethink-beliefs-gmos/20444059/.

18. Daley, Cynthia A., Amber Abbott, Patrick S. Doyle, Glenn A. Nader, and Stephanie Larson. "A Review of Fatty Acid Profiles and Antioxidant Content in Grass-fed and Grain-fed Beef." *Nutrition Journal.* BioMed Central, n.d. Web. 24 Feb. 2015. http://www.ncbi.nlm.nih.gov/pmc/articles/PMC2846864/.

19. Sarah K. Gebauer, Jean-Michel Chardigny, Marianne Uhre Jakobsen, Benoît Lamarche, Adam L. Lock, Spencer D. Proctor and David J. Baer. "Effects of Ruminant Trans Fatty Acids on Cardiovascular Disease and Cancer: A Comprehensive Review of Epidemiological, Clinical, and Mechanistic Studies." *Advances in Nutrition.* N.p., 2011.

20. "Diabetes." *Effect of Fructose Overfeeding and Fish Oil Administration on Hepatic De Novo Lipogenesis and Insulin Sensitivity in Healthy Men.* Web. 24 Feb. 2015. http://diabetes.diabetesjournals.org/content/54/7/1907.short.

21. " *National Center for Biotechnology Information.* U.S. National Library of Medicine, n.d. Web. 24 Feb. 2015. http://www.ncbi.nlm.nih.gov/pubmed/20219526.

22. " *National Center for Biotechnology Information.* U.S. National Library of Medicine, n.d. Web. 24 Feb. 2015. http://www.ncbi.nlm.nih.gov/pubmed/24558989.

23. *National Center for Biotechnology Information.* U.S. National Library of Medicine, n.d. Web. 24 Feb. 2015. http://www.ncbi.nlm.nih.gov/pubmed/24366371.

24. *National Center for Biotechnology Information.* U.S. National Library of Medicine, n.d. Web. 24 Feb. 2015. http://www.ncbi.nlm.nih.gov/pubmed/23594708.

25. "Trans Fatty Acids and Coronary Heart Disease—NEJM." New England Journal of Medicine. N.p., n.d. Web. 24 Feb. 2015. http://www.nejm.org/doi/full/10.1056/NEJM199906243402511.

26. *National Center for Biotechnology Information.* U.S. National Library of Medicine, n.d. Web. 24 Feb. 2015. http://www.ncbi.nlm.nih.gov/pubmed/11893781.

27. "Dodd-Frank Wall Steet Reform 291 in the Last Year." *Federal Register.* Web. 24 Feb. 2015. https://www.federalregister.gov/articles/1999/11/17/99–29537/food-labeling-trans-fatty-acids-in-nutrition-labeling-nutrient-content-claims-and-health-claims.

28. "Journal of Nutrition." *The Safety Evaluation of Monosodium Glutamate.* Web. 24 Feb. 2015. http://jn.nutrition.org/content/130/4/1049S.full.

29. Soffritti, M. "First Experimental Demonstration of the Multipotential Carcinogenic Effects of Aspartame Administered in the Feed to Sprague-Dawley Rats." *National Center for Biotechnology Information.* U.S. National Library of Medicine, 2006.

30. Warner, Melanie. "The Lowdown on Sweet?" *The New York Times.* The New York Times, 11 Feb. 2006. http://www.nytimes.com/2006/02/12/business/yourmoney/12sweet.html?pagewanted=all&_r=0.

31. "Specific Sugar Molecule Causes Growth of Cancer Cells." *ScienceDaily.*

32. Cary, R., S. Dobson, and E. Ball. *Azodicarbonamide.* Geneva: World Health Organization, 1999. Web.

33. *National Center for Biotechnology Information.* U.S. National Library of Medicine, n.d. Web. 02 Mar. 2015.

34. "Review of Harmful Gastrointestinal Effects of Carrageenan in Animal Experiments." *National Center for Biotechnology Information.* U.S. National Library of Medicine.

35. Gheldof N1, Wang XH, Engeseth NJ. "Identification and Quantification of Antioxidant Components of Honeys from Various Floral Sources." *National Center for Biotechnology Information.* U.S. National Library of Medicine, Oct. 2002.

36. "Natural Honey Lowers Plasma Glucose, C-reactive Protein, Homocysteine, and Blood Lipids in Healthy, Diabetic, and Hyperlipidemic Subjects: Comparison with Dextrose and Sucrose." *National Center for Biotechnology Information.* U.S. National Library of Medicine, 2004.

37. Chan, Paul, Brian Tomlinson, Yi-Jen Chen, Ju-Chi Liu, Ming-Hsiung Hsieh, and Juei-Tang Cheng. "A Double-blind Placebo-controlled Study of the Effectiveness and Tolerability of Oral Stevioside in Human Hypertension." *British Journal of Clinical Pharmacology.* Blackwell Science Inc, Sept. 2000.

38. Søren Gregersena, Per B Jeppesena, Jens J Holstb, Kjeld Hermansen. "Antihyperglycemic Effects of Stevioside in Type 2 Diabetic Subjects." *Science Direct.*

39. "Xylitol and Caries Prevention—Is It a Magic Bullet?" *Nature.com.* Nature Publishing Group, 2003.

40. "The Effects of Xylitol on the Secretion of Insulin and Gastric Inhibit." *Ory Polypeptide in Man and Rats.* N.p., 01 June 1982.

41. Noda K, Nakayama K, Oku T. "Serum Glucose and Insulin Levels and Erythritol Balance after Oral Administration of Erythritol in Healthy Subjects." *European Journal of Clinical Nutrition.* N.p., Apr. 1994

42. "Colas, but Not Other Carbonated Beverages, Are Associated with Low Bone Mineral Density in Older Women: The Framingham Osteoporosis Study." *National Center for Biotechnology Information.* U.S. National

Library of Medicine.

43. "Relation between Consumption of Sugar-sweetened Drinks and Childhood Obesity: A Prospective, Observational Analysis." *National Center for Biotechnology Information.* U.S. National Library of Medicine.

44. Kumar GS, Pan L, Park S, Lee-Kwan SH, Onufrak S, Blanck HM. "Sugar-sweetened Beverage Consumption among Adults—18 States, 2012." *National Center for Biotechnology Information.* U.S. National Library of Medicine, Aug. 2014.

45. Choi HK, Willett W, Curhan G. "Fructose-Rich Beverages and Risk of Gout in Women." *JAMA.* 2010; 304:2270–8.

46. Choi HK, Curhan G. "Soft Drinks, Fructose Consumption and the Risk of Gout in Men: Prospective Cohort Study." *BMJ.* 2008; 336:309–12.

47. Dann AB, Hontela A. "Triclosan: Environmental Exposure, Toxicity and Mechanisms of Action." *National Center for Biotechnology Information.* U.S. National Library of Medicine, May 2011.

48. "Maternal Exposure to Triclosan Impairs Thyroid Homeostasis and Female Pubertal Development in Wistar Rat Offspring." *National Center for Biotechnology Information.* U.S. National Library of Medicine.

49. Robin E. Dodson, Marcia Nishioka, Laurel J. Standley, Laura J. Perovich, Julia Green Brody, and Ruthann A. Rudel. "EHP—Endocrine Disruptors and Asthma-Associated Chemicals in Consumer Products." *EHP.* N.p., July 2012.

50. Rule KL, Ebbett VR, Vikesland PJ "Formation of chloroform and chlorinated organics by free-chlorine-mediated oxidation of triclosan." 2005.

51. Geens T, Neels H, Covaci A. *Distribution of bisphenol-A, triclosan and n-nonylphenol in human adipose tissue, liver and brain. Chemosphere,* Environ. Sci. Technol. 39 (9): 3176–85. doi:10.1021/es048943.

52. Committee on the Assessment of Asthma and Indoor Air, Division of Health Promotion and Disease Prevention, Institute of Medicine "Clearing the Air: Asthma and Indoor Air Exposures." *Institute of Medicine.* 2000.

53. "Body Burden: The Pollution in Newborns." *Environmental Working Group.* http://www.ewg.org/research/body-burden-pollution-newborns

54. "The Trouble with Sunscreen Chemicals." Http://www.ewg.

org/2014sunscreen/the-trouble-with-sunscreen-chemicals/. (n.d.): n. pag. Web.

55. "Scientific Committee on Consumer Safety." *OPINION ON Quaternium-15 (cis-isomer)* (2011): n. pag. Web.

56. CA EPA. "California Dry Cleaning Industry Technical Assessment Report." N.p., Oct. 2005.

57. Mnif, Wissem, Aziza Ibn Hadj Hassine, Aicha Bouaziz, Aghleb Bartegi, Olivier Thomas, and Benoit Roig. "Effect of Endocrine Disruptor Pesticides: A Review." *International Journal of Environmental Research and Public Health.* Molecular Diversity Preservation International (MDPI).

Acknowledgements

I find it strange sometimes how life can deliver us along a path that leads us to remarkable people and life-changing situations. We moved in next door to an Integrative Nutrition Health Coach back in 2009. If I hadn't met my neighbor, I wouldn't be in this place right now of helping others and sharing my passion for healthy living. Thanks, Amy Butchko, for opening your door and letting me in.

Thank you to my amazing tribe of clients who inspire me daily. Your incredible life-changing results are what keep me going every day. I am blessed to be able to support each and every one of you.

Thank you to my parents for supporting me and believing in me.

To my dear friends at the Four Seasons Community: you all have inspired me and I can't thank you enough for your continued support. It's been so fun teaching you and supporting you toward better health.

Thank you to my small army of recipe testers who volunteered to try my recipes. Thank you for helping me make this book available for anyone who wants to get in the kitchen.

Thank you to Pam for giving me your opinions and help. They are very much appreciated.

And last, but not least, thank you to my amazing husband for supporting me, believing in me and always being there.

About the Author

Meet Cindy Santa Ana

Cindy is an Integrative Nutrition Health Coach and founder of Unlock Better Health. She is deeply passionate about inspiring her clients to reach their ideal weight, increase their energy and live a healthy balanced lifestyle while juggling their career and personal life.

Her articles have been featured in Fitlife.tv, Club Take Back Your Health, *Woman's World*, and The DC Ladies.

When she's not teaching cooking classes or presenting workshops on health, you can find her gardening or playing with her kids in her Northern Virginia backyard.

To find out more, visit her website at UnlockBetterHealth.com, and sign up for your free Health Strategy session today.

42388718R00121

Made in the USA
Lexington, KY
19 June 2015